Ayurvedic Herbology-EAST & WEST

The Practical Guide to Ayurvedic Herbal Medicine

Vishnu Dass

MOTILAL BANARSIDASS PUBLISHERS
PRIVATE LIMITED • DELHI

*First Indian Edition : **Delhi, 2017***

Published in arrangement with
LOTUS PRESS
P.O. Box 325, Twin Lakes, WI 53181 USA

ISBN: 978-81-208-4099-7

Also available at

MOTILAL BANARSIDASS
41 U.A., Bungalow Road, Jawahar Nagar, Delhi 110 007
8 Mahalaxmi Chamber, 22 Bhulabhai Desai Road, Mumbai 400 026
203 Royapettah High Road, Mylapore, Chennai 600 004
236, 9th Main III Block, Jayanagar, Bangalore 560 011
8 Camac Street, Kolkata 700 017
Ashok Rajpath, Patna 800 004
Chowk, Varanasi 221 001

DISCLAIMER

The information contained in this book is provided as a reference and by no means intended to diagnose, treat, or prescribe. This book should not be used as a substitute for professional medical care or treatment and the reader is a advised to consult with a health care professional before taking any herbs or herbal supplements.

FOR SALE IN SOUTH ASIA ONLY

Library of Congress Number : 2013950062

Published by
Motilal Banarsidass Publishers Private Limited
www.mlbd.com • mlbd@mlbd.com
Printed by Gopsons Papers Private Limited

Contents

Part IV: Ayurvedic Materia Medica

Medicinal Herbs: East and West

PART V: APPENDICES

ACKNOWLEDGEMENTS

I want to give special thanks to my beloved teacher Dr. Vasant Lad, for sharing with me the ancient science of Ayurveda. Without his generosity and wisdom, this book would not have been possible.

I would also like to give many thanks to my editor Yol Swan, for her keen eye for detail and her encouragement and support during all phases of the creation of this book.

Thanks also to Aaron Ananta Staengl, for providing me with his illustration of Lord Dhanvantari.

I am also grateful for everyone at Lotus Press for making the publishing of this book possible.

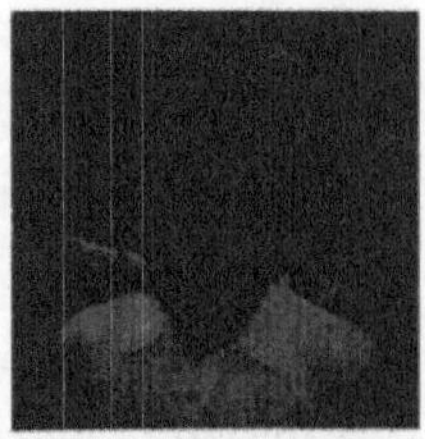

Vishnu Dass
Blue Lotus Ayurveda
Asheville, NC
Ph. 828-713-4266
Email: clinic@bluelotusayurveda.com
www.bluelotusayurveda.com

AYURVEDIC HERBOLOGY: EAST AND WEST

An Ayurvedic Approach to Medicinal Herbs

Foreword

When Vishnu Dass was my student, he was a very spiritual, attentive, and dedicated student and always worked with great sincerity. Now he has been in practice for a number of years, and his horizon of wisdom continues to expand and to be enhanced. He has taken his wise experience and written a guide to herbology based on Ayurvedic principles.

This wonderful, practical book is one of the masterpieces of Ayurvedic herbology work. He has put a lot of effort into this and his dedication, devotion, and commitment to Ayurveda and to his teacher is very beautiful. He has explained in simple but direct terms the Ayurvedic approach to health, herbal medicine, and materia medica. Plus, he has elaborated on Ayurvedic history and philosophy and of Ayurvedic principles, and concepts regarding the five elements, three doshas, and the subdoshas. He has wonderfully blended these philosophies into a direct application of herbology.

He has given a most practical approach of Ayurvedic herbology providing the action and classification of each herb including rasa, virya, vipaka and prabhav, and each botanical, Ayurvedic, and Sanskrit name.

He also covers the western concepts of herbology, including western pharmacological actions such as alterative, anti-inflammatory, anti-microbial, anti-pyretic, and diaphoretics. Additionally, he has presented these functions for Ayurvedic herbs.

This book breathes the life of practical Ayurvedic principles, methodology, pharmaceutical and pharmacological actions. For example, key points in Ayurvedic herbology are the timing of taking herbs and their dosages, and he has elaborated on that quite effectively. He also expounds upon the Ayurvedic principles of formulation according to dosha and disease as well as classical herbal preparation techniques.

Historically, Ayurvedic medicinal preparations looked for methods to preserve the effectiveness of herbs that would match that of fresh herbs. The rasa, virya, and vipaka of fresh herbs are readily available, but the ancient rishis looked for methods to use with dry herbs also. To have a preparation that could be as effective as swarasa, fresh juice, this text advises you to take one part of the dry herb to two parts water and soak these overnight. Squeeze this mixture through cheesecloth and the results are similar to the fresh juice, a modification of swarasa.

Another method is kvatha, a decoction by volume of one part herb and 16 parts water, boiled until it yields ¼ part as a decoction. The rishis were trying to preserve herbs, but even stored decoctions and swarasas only last a short time. The next stage of longer lasting herbal medicines was to cook the decoction with equal quantities of oil or ghee, creating medicated oils and ghees that would last for years. This is the natural way of preservation in Ayurveda, without chemical preservatives.

In their continued quest for immortality, the rishis next produced gutika and vatika, pill forms of herbs. Their crowning achievement was siddha kalpa or rasa shastra. In siddha kalpa, they incorporated mercury, sulphur, silver, gold, copper, tin, zinc, and iron bhasmas (ash) into medicines that heal the very essence of the human body. The rishis found that mixing this bhasma with herbal compounds caused them to be effective indefinitely and that even very small doses can have profound, positive results. Bhasmas do their job and leave the body through the urine, feces, and sweat.

To use such heavy metals, they must be made safe for human consumption, to be 'humanized.' To do this, they heat the metal until it is red hot and then dip it in sesame oil , then cow's urine, cow's milk, cow's yogurt, cow's buttermilk, cow's butter, and finally in ghee. Each step is performed seven times, one for each tissue. This absorbs the toxic poisonous properties of the heavy metal and it becomes humanized. This humanized form is burned into ash, which is the bhasma used in medicine. There are three important tests of proper processing for the safety and purity of the ash. A pinch of the bhasma should float on the surface of water; that test is varitaratva. This means it can easily pass through the cytoplasm of the cell and into the rasa dhatu, the serum and blood plasma. The specific gravity of the ash is less than water and can pass through the surface tension and surface angle of the plasma. Next, take the bhasma and rub it between the index finger and thumb. It should spread into the ridges of the finger, the fingerprints. This test, rekhaagamitra, means the bhasma will easily pass through the capillaries. Finally, apunarbhava; you should not see any trace of the metal because it is pulverized. This is the ancient science of Ayurvedic metallurgy and alchemy. Metal becomes pure energy, vibrational medicine.

Vishnu Dass has covered many subtle topics in this quite scholarly work. In a true sense, this is an integrated work, both for eastern and western herbalists, who can use this knowledge for healing and creating effective herbal products. It is a thorough explanation of

Ayurvedic techniques, which add a new dimension to the western herbalist practice. By including the Ayurvedic rasa, virya, vipaka, and prabhava for the western herbs, he enables practitioners to expand the horizon of their experience. This book is a practical guide, both for students and practitioners, with clear directions to formulate individualistic formulas, including constitutional and vikruti solutions.

Vasant Lad, B.A.M. & S., M.A.Sc.
Ayurvedic Physician
Albuquerque
June 2012

Part I:
An Introduction to Ayurveda

Philosophical and Historical Background

The Spiritual and Holistic Foundation of Ayurveda

Ayurveda is one of the oldest systems of health in the world. Dating back more than 5000 years, it finds its roots in ancient India. It is a complete system of medicine that aims to prevent imbalance, maintain a high quality of life, and increase the longevity of the individual. In Sanskrit *ayus* means "life" and *veda* refers to a system of "knowledge" or "wisdom" (and "teachings"), so Ayurveda is often referred to as the "Science of Life." According to the *Charaka Samhita*, one of the main ancient texts on Ayurveda, life is the combination of the body, sense organs, mind, and individual soul. In other words, it is the integration of body, mind, and consciousness. In this sense, Ayurveda is a truly holistic system that embraces all aspects of human nature in their interaction with the environment and the laws of creation. It is also a science of self-knowledge that provides guidelines to help prevent disease and maintain health through self-awareness and discipline. Furthermore, it is the art of living in harmony with nature.

Health and disease in Ayurveda can only be understood when all aspects of life—from the physical to the mental and emotional, as well as the spiritual—are taken into consideration. Each and every part of the body-mind complex has to be perceived in its intimate relationship with the whole. Ayurvedic medicines and therapies are meant to support and promote the natural ability of the body-mind complex to heal itself. Ultimately, we are each responsible for our actions and well-being. This is why it is so important to take an active part in the healing process, while rediscovering and learning to trust our inner intelligence. In this sense, Ayurveda—with its down-to-earth, common sense approach—can be an empowering tool to regain control over our health.

Ayurveda is a spiritual science in itself, grounded in the rich philosophical and spiritual traditions of India. As a branch of the Vedas, it is a stream of the knowledge passed down from generation to generation since time immemorial, much in the same way as Vedic literature and scriptures were. According to the *Charaka Samhita*, the knowledge of Ayurveda is eternal and is revealed in each of the cycles of creation and destruction of the universe.

One of the main philosophical systems that serves as the foundation for both Ayurveda and the *Ashtanga* (Eight Limb) yoga system is *Samkhya*. Founded by the sage Kapila, *Samkhya* philosophy states that this entire creation evolved out of the interaction of *Purusha*, or pure consciousness, and *Prakruti* (also *Prakriti*), or primordial matter. *Purusha* is beyond all attributes such as name, form, or quality, and is the witness of creation. It is the inner self in all. *Prakruti* is the creative potential, the one that manifests as the many and has color, form, and all other attributes, but is unconscious and requires the influence of *Purusha* to animate it. All activity within creation—from the unmanifest, or latent seeds of potential, down to the gross matter—is guided by the presence of *Purusha*, in the same manner that an iron wheel is turned by the invisible influence of a magnet.

The universal *Prakruti* is "the first cause" from which the entire creation unfolds. *Prakruti* has three basic qualities or *gunas*: *Sattwa, rajas*, and *tamas*. *Sattwa* is associated with the quality of light or purity, *rajas* with the energy of action, and *tamas* with that of inertia and gross matter. These qualities exist in perfect balance within the unmanifest aspect of *Prakruti*. When this balance is disturbed, the entire creation develops, like ripples upon the waters of the cosmos. It is in this field of manifestation that *Purusha* has the ability to experience itself and the world, as well as to seek liberation from experience and become fully Self-realized, which is the ultimate goal of human life.

The first expression of *Prakruti* is *Mahat*, or the cosmic intellect that has the nature of the pure "I am." In this state, *Prakruti* receives the light of *Purusha* and becomes conscious of consciousness. Just as a seed contains every aspect of a fruit, plant, or tree within it, *Mahat* contains all of the creative potential of *Prakruti*. On the level of the individual soul, *Mahat* appears as the individual intellect, or *buddhi*, which is the discriminating faculty of the mind.

Buddhi manifests from the *sattwic* aspect of *Prakruti* and has the ability to reflect the light of *Purusha*, in a similar manner as a still pool of water reflects the light of the moon. During the evolutionary phase, *buddhi* loses discrimination between its real nature (pure consciousness) and the unreal (the ever changing form of *Prakruti*), and manifests as *ahamkara*, the individual consciousness, or ego. This false "I-sense" perceives itself as separate from the whole and takes on the form of the fluctuating thoughts in the mind. Since the mind serves the interests of the ego, we all experience the world according to our own impressions, thought patterns, and projections.

Obviously, how we view the world largely depends on the predominant nature of our mind and our inner tendencies, as these constantly color our perceptions.

This is why, according to Ayurveda, all disease has a mental, emotional, and physical component. All impressions and tendencies in the mind permeate our needs, drives, habits, relationships, addictions, and so on. Thought waves and impressions are constantly expressing themselves through the body. For instance, if we love ourselves and believe that we deserve to be loved, we will project those beliefs through our attitude, habits, relationships, and general state of health. On the other hand, suppressed or unresolved emotions will cause imbalance. In the same manner as bad food combining causes *ama* (toxins), because the body cannot properly process certain food combinations, unresolved (or "unprocessed") emotions and impressions can also cause mental *ama*, which will eventually manifest as disease. This is where Ayurveda stresses that yogic practices and meditation are invaluable to quiet the mind and remove the emotional garbage we all carry, while increasing the flow of *prana*, or vital energy, to nourish all aspects of the body-mind complex.

For the ancient Indian *rishis*, or seers of truth, the concept of being separate from nature did not exist. All that was outside also manifested within, be it the planets and stars, or the mountains, rivers, and valleys. Through their close relationship with nature and their earnest search for the truth within, they conveyed the wisdom of how to live in harmony with the laws of nature. These sages closely observed and learned from their surroundings, and understood that every living thing helps to maintain the delicate balance of nature. All living things have a place and a particular role to play, just as every cell of our body has a specific function and is in constant communication with every other cell. The *rishis* also understood that the health of the one meant the health of the whole, and vice versa.

It is obvious that all the great technological advancements of the modern civilized world have brought us far from the simplicity of nature and have disrupted the harmony and balance at the global level as well. The current general disregard for nature is a reflection of the collective state of the human race. The damming of the rivers can be likened to the hardening and blockage of arteries, the lack of rain to the drying up of tissues and vital fluids, and environmental pollutants to the accumulated toxins in the body. The global dilemma is truly an individual one. If contact is lost with nature, disharmony will prevail and reflect in our surroundings.

At the same time, many of the world's ancient spiritual traditions are now spreading across the planet to benefit humanity. The wisdom of Ayurveda has begun to span the globe, being needed now as much as ever before. It is hard to create a change globally if we cannot take responsibility for our own health and well-being as individuals. To change the state of the planet we need to start by changing our patterns, habits, and lifestyle, and embrace and respect nature as we move through the different cycles, seasons, and phases of life. Ayurveda provides practical guidelines to help us maintain a healthy balance with our environment and restore our connection with the whole.

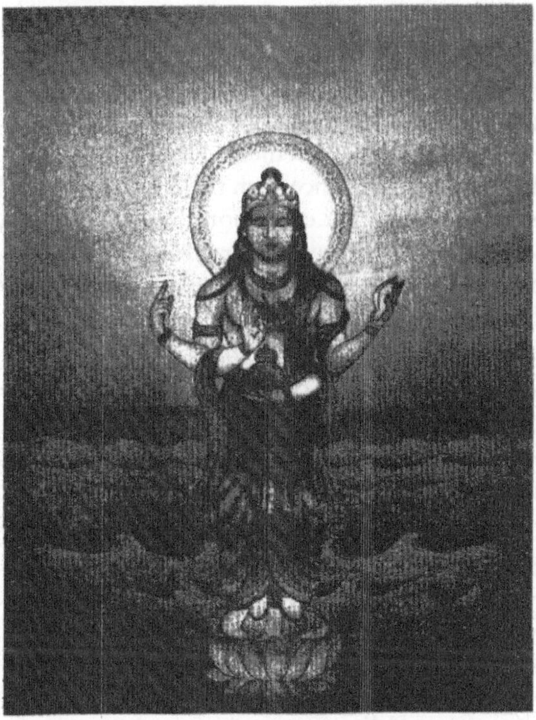

Lord Dhanvantari, Divine Father of Ayurveda

Lord Dhanvantari is known as the father of Ayurveda, since he was the first divine incarnation to impart its wisdom amongst humans. He first appeared during the great churning of the cosmic ocean of milk (*Samudra manthan*) to deliver *amrit* (ambrosia) to the demigods. The churning of the ocean of milk is a famous episode in the *Puranas* that represents the spiritual endeavor of a person to achieve Self-realization through concentration of mind, withdrawal of the senses, control of all desires, austerities, and asceticism. It is celebrated in India every twelve years in the festival known as *Kumbha Mela*. The following story about Lord Dhanvantari is related in the *Srimad Bhagavatam*.

Indra, the great leader of the *devas* (demigods), was riding on his elephant when he came across the sage Durvasa Muni. Seeing the great demigod, Durvasa offered him a special garland that had been blessed by Sri, another manifestation of Laxmi, the Goddess of Abundance. Indra accepted the garland nonchalantly and put it on the trunk of his elephant, but the animal swiftly tossed it on the ground. Durvasa Muni was very upset by this display of disrespect, and in anger cursed Indra and all the *devas* to be bereft of all strength, energy, and fortune right then and there.

Taking advantage of this situation, the *asuras* (demons) attacked the demigods, killing many of them, and slowly gaining control of the universe. Indra and the other *devas* rushed to Brahma for help. Brahma suggested they bring their predicament to Lord Vishnu, who in turn advised them to seek alliance with the *asuras* to churn the ocean of milk together for the nectar of immortality. The demigods agreed only because Lord Vishnu promised that He would make sure they alone would obtain the nectar and recover their strength and power to defeat the demons.

Both *devas* and *asuras* proceeded to churn the ocean of milk, and it was such an arduous task that Lord Vishnu had to appear in many forms to help them with this process and prevent it from going nowhere. He even showed up as Lord Vishnu himself, sitting on top of the mountain to infuse Indra and his companions with energy.

All kinds of herbs were cast into the ocean. The churning first produced a deadly poison (*halahala*) that Lord Shiva had to swallow, being the only one who would not be affected by it. Many other objects and beings slowly emerged from the ocean as well, including Kamadhenu (the wish fulfilling cow), Ucchaisrava (the white horse), Airavata (the white elephant), Kaustubhamani (a rare diamond), Kalpavriksha (the wish fulfilling tree), and Sri Laxmi, the Goddess of Wealth, who after being worshipped by all *devas* and *asuras*, was finally reunited with her husband Lord Vishnu, after many ages of separation.

As the churning continued, Lord Dhanvantari appeared. He was young and strongly built, his chest was very broad and his complexion bluish black. He had muscular arms, reddish eyes, and moved like a lion. He was clad in bright yellow, his curly hair was anointed with oil, and he wore shining earrings made of pearl. As he emerged, he was holding a conch, leeches, healing herbs, a *chakra* (one of the divine weapons of Lord Vishṇu's), and the long sought pot of ambrosia, for which he is also called *Sudha Pani* ("carrying nectar"). The *asuras*, greedy after all things, realized right away that the container was full of nectar, and snatched it from him.

However, the demons immediately started quarreling about which of them would drink the nectar first, grabbing the pot from one another, and behaving like thieves. Seeing how busy they were fighting with each other, Lord Vishnu didn't miss the opportunity to trick them. He appeared as Mohini, a beautiful woman who fascinated the demons, recovered the nectar from them, and distributed it only among the demigods. As soon as the *devas* drank it, they were invigorated with energy and defeated the demons. After worshipping Lord Vishnu and Sri Laxmi, they resumed their position in the heavens. At the time, Lord Vishnu foretold that Lord Dhanvantari would appear again in the world to teach men the science of Ayurveda.

Later on, Lord Indra, seeing humanity so afflicted by pain and disease, pleaded with Lord Dhanvantari to descend into the material world and teach Ayurveda to the human race. At that time, the King Dirghatamas of Kashi (Benares) was performing severe austerities and offering them to Lord Dhanvantari, in the hopes that he would grant him a son. The Lord appeared and offered a boon to the king, so Dirghatamas asked Him to be born as his own son. The Lord replied that he would.

Soon after, Lord Dhanvantari was born in the royal household of Kashi and eventually became the king. Even as a young boy he had ascetic tendencies, was extremely disciplined, and performed severe austerities. He taught Ayurveda orally to the sages and *rishis* (seers) who became his disciples. His teachings are recorded in the *Agni Purana*, as well as through the teachings of his disciples Sushruta, Pauskalavata, Aurabha, Vaitarana, and others.

It is written in the scriptures that, "One who remembers the name of Dhanvantari can be released from all disease." Lord Dhanvantari is worshipped all over India as the God of Medicine. Even today, two days before Diwali, the Festival of Lights, people remember and honor him. At dusk, a lamp pointing toward North by North-East is lit at the doorstep of the house to welcome Lord Dhanvantari for health and happiness in life.

Brief Historical Overview

The knowledge of Ayurveda was originally passed down from masters to their disciples in an unbroken oral tradition, and although different Vedic texts mention certain aspects of Ayurveda, it is mainly considered a branch of the *Atharva Veda*. Eventually, it was refined into a complete system of medicine and in time two schools of Ayurveda developed: The Atreya school of physicians and the Dhanvantari school of surgeons. These two schools transformed Ayurveda into the medical system we know today.

Ayurveda became a respected system of medicine between the 8th and 6th century BC, and people from many countries attended Indian Ayurvedic schools to learn it. This is probably how Ayurvedic principles and concepts were integrated into other medical systems, including the Tibetan, Chinese, Greek, Egyptian, and Persian. India's Silk Road (the trade route between Asia, the Middle East, and Europe) also provided a link between those cultures and the exchange of medical and scientific knowledge.

After the many invasions to India, Ayurveda lost ground. Ayurvedic colleges were closed and books destroyed by various conquerors. The last Ayurvedic universities were closed during the British rule of India. Yet the knowledge continued to be transmitted from masters to students in oral form, as it had for centuries before. Finally, Ayurveda reemerged during the 1920's, and universities were rebuilt with funding from the Indian government. Nowadays, Ayurveda is becoming increasingly recognized in the West as one of the most natural, holistic, and effective forms of herbal medicine and health care in the world.

The Eight Branches of Ayurveda

Around 1500 B.C., the two main schools of Ayurveda classified the medical system into eight branches:

1. Kaya Chikitsa (internal medicine) related to the body, mind, and spirit as a whole. It considered internal and external causes of disease and included the pathogenesis of disease, tridosha and doshic imbalance, botanical classification of Materia Medica, and methods such as Panchakarma for cleansing and cellular rejuvenation.
2. Shalakya Tantra (medicine for the ears, nose, and throat) focused on the ears, nose, and throat, and discussed both therapeutics and surgical procedures.
3. Vishagara-Vairodh Tantra (toxicology) included aspects of air

and water pollution, toxins in general, and epidemics, as well as symptom assessment and therapeutic methods.

4. Kaumara Bhritya (pediatrics) addressed prenatal and postpartum care of both baby and mother. It also included methods of conception, midwifery, and childhood diseases.
5. Shalya Tantra (surgery) focused on sophisticated surgical methods, used only as a last resort.
6. Bhuta Vidya (psychiatry) dealt specifically with disturbances of the mind, including demonic possession, through the use of herbs, therapies, and spiritual practices like pranayama (breathing techniques) and mantra (words of power).
7. Vajikarana (aphrodisiacs) referred to sterility, infertility, and problems of both male and female reproductive systems, as well as the transmutation of sexual energy for spiritual purposes.
8. Rasayana (rejuvenation) discussed the prevention of disease and the promotion of longevity.

The Main Ayurvedic Texts

The knowledge of Ayurveda was reorganized and compiled into three main treatises that are still used today by both students and practitioners: The *Charaka Samhita,* which grew from the Atreya school of physicians and is considered the most important of all the ancient texts, covered all aspects of clinical practice, including physiology, anatomy, etiology, pathogenesis, symptoms and signs of disease, methodology of diagnosis, treatment, and prescription, prevention, and longevity. The *Sushruta Samhita,* which came from the Dhanvantari school of surgeons, covered surgical equipment, classification of abscesses, burns, fractures, wounds, amputation, plastic and rectal surgery, and included anatomical discussions of bones, joints, nerves, organs, blood vessels, vital points, and major human systems.

The *Ashtanga Hridayam*, written in verse by Vagbhata, consisted of a synthesis of earlier Ayurvedic texts, with a focus on internal medicine (*kaya chikitsa*). Another work associated with the same author (although often referred to as Vagbhata II) is the *Ashtanga Samgraha*, which was written in a mixture of verse and prose, and contained much of the same material in a more discursive form.

The works of Charaka, Sushruta, and Vagbhata are reverentially called the *Vriddha Trayi*, which can be translated as "the Triad of Ancients," or *Brhat Trayi*, which means "the Greater Triad." The *Madhava Nidana*, *Sharngadhara Samhita*, and *Bhava Prakasha* are the lesser three classic Ayurvedic texts that assumed a position of authority during the 1st, 15th, and 16th centuries. These texts show the profound knowledge of the body-mind complex as well as the rich botanical and mineral resources of India that Ayurvedic physicians and surgeons have had throughout history.

Main Ayurvedic Principles and Concepts

Five Element Theory and *Gunas*, the Qualities of Nature

The ancient *rishis* viewed that the entire creation is a play of the *Pancha Mahabhutas*, or five great elements: Earth, water, fire, air, and ether (or space). Ayurveda shares with yoga philosophy the view that a human being is the combination of the five great elements plus the immaterial self.

Every substance is made up of these five elements and can be classified according to its predominant element. For example, a mountain is predominantly made up of the earth element, so it is classified as earth, yet it also contains water, fire, air, and ether in smaller amounts. Below is a brief description of each element.

Earth: *Prithvi*

Earth represents the solid state of matter. It manifests stability, permanence, and rigidity. In our body, the parts such as bones, teeth, cells, and tissues are manifestations of the earth element. Earth is considered a stable substance.

Water: *Apas*

Water characterizes change and represents the liquid state. Water is necessary for the survival of all living things. A large part of the human body is made up of water. Our blood, lymph, and other fluids move between our cells and through our vessels, bringing energy, carrying away wastes, regulating temperature, moving disease fighting cells, and taking hormonal information from one area to another. Water is a substance without stability.

Fire: *Tejas*

Fire is the element that transforms solids into liquids or gas and back. In other words, it possesses the power to change the state of any substance. Within the body, this energy binds the atoms together. Fire transforms food into energy: It converts food into fat (stored energy) and muscle. It also creates the impulses of nervous reactions, including our feelings and even our thought processes. Fire is considered a form without substance.

Air: *Vayu*

Air is the gaseous form of matter that is mobile and dynamic. Within the body, air (as oxygen) is the basis for all energy transfer reactions. It is a key element required for fire to burn. Air is existence without form.

Ether: *Akasha*

Ether is the ground of all existence from where the other elements arise. It is the space in which everything happens. So it is simultaneously the source of all matter and the space in which it exists. Ether is the distances that separate matter. The chief characteristic of ether is sound, where sound represents the entire spectrum of vibration.

The Three *Doshas*

In Ayurveda the key to understanding the individual constitution, or *prakruti*, is the concept of *tridosha*. *Tridosha* theory defines the three *doshas* or fundamental principles that govern the functions of the body on the physical, mental, and emotional levels. Each of these psycho-physiological principles is made up primarily of two of the five elements. In other words, the five elements manifesting as the *doshas* animate all living beings. We can infer the existence of the *doshas* through the various functions they govern in the body-mind complex. In balance, they maintain normal functions, and out of balance they promote the disease process. These three energies are known as *vata*, *pitta*, and *kapha*.

We all have the qualities of all three *doshas* in our constitution, but often one or two *doshas* are predominant, while the others remain secondary. Ayurveda identifies seven main constitutional types with innumerable variations, depending upon the percentage of each *dosha* in the individual constitution, as well as their unique qualitative expression in the body. Below is a general description of the main characteristics of the three *doshas*.

Vata Dosha

Mainly composed of ether (space) and air, *vata* is the subtle energy associated with movement. It regulates all activity in the body—from the physiological to the mental and psychological aspects. It governs the equilibrium of the tissues and the functions of respiration, circulation, elimination, speech, pulsation of the heart, and neuron impulses, as well as the movement of vital fluids and nutrients to every cell of the body. *Vata* also moves the other two *doshas*, so any aggravation of this *dosha* can in turn bring imbalances related to *pitta* and *kapha*. Furthermore, *vata* is responsible for *prana*, the vital essence that maintains the life of the body. When *vata* leaves the body, life ceases.

The colon is the main site of *vata*, but it is also present in the nervous system as neuron impulses, in the ears, pelvic cavity, low back, sacrum, thighs, joints, and skin. When *vata* is increased, there may be signs and symptoms connected to these locations.

In its natural state, *vata* promotes creativity and flexibility. Out of balance, *vata* can give rise to emotional disturbances like fear, anxiety, and restlessness, as well as abnormal movements (twitching, tremors, tics, spasms, convulsions, and so on). When disturbed, it can also create dryness, constipation, flatulence, abdominal distention and discomfort, loss of strength, diminished sensory acuity, fatigue, insomnia, and dark skin discolorations. *Vata* is often the main etiological factor in cases of degenerative and neurological disorders.

Characteristics of *Vata*

Physically, *vata* people have light body frames, under developed muscles, and predominant joints, veins, and muscle tendons. *Vata* types tend to be slightly underweight and often feel cold, especially their hands and feet. They love warm weather and sunbathing. Their appetite and digestion is often variable and they are prone to experiencing gas, bloating, and malabsorption. They have a tendency toward constipation, dryness, and cracking of the skin due to the dry and rough qualities of *vata*.

Vata individuals tend to be either tall or short and may have crooked or protruded teeth. They tan easily and have a darker complexion than the other *doshas*. The eyes may be small, dark, and active, or restless and perhaps sunken. Their hair is typically dry, curly, frizzy, thin, or scanty and their nails brittle or cracked.

Mentally, *vata* individuals are often active, easily excited, creative, alert, and quick to act out of impulse. They think a lot and tend to give way to worry, anxiety, and fear. They understand quickly but tend to forget quickly as well. They are daydreamers with vivid imaginations, talkative, nervous and tend to fidget, fiddle, and bite their nails. Due to their active nature, they will create tasks to prevent boredom from setting in. *Vata* types may experience light and interrupted sleep.

Vata qualities are dry, light, cold, rough, subtle, mobile (erratic), clear, and astringent. These qualities translate into the makeup of the *vata* individual, as shown in the chart of *vata* attributes below.

Qualities in the *Vata* Individual

Attributes	Constitutional Manifestations
Dry (*ruksha*)	Dry skin, hair, lips, and tongue; dry colon, tendency toward constipation; hoarse voice.
Light (*laghu*)	Light muscles, bones, thin body frame; light, scanty sleep; tendency to be underweight.
Cold (*shita*)	Cold hands and feet; poor circulation; hates cold and loves hot; stiffness of muscles.
Rough (*khara*)	Rough or cracked skin, nails, hair, teeth, hands, and feet; cracking joints.
Subtle (*sukshma*)	Subtle fear, anxiety, and insecurity; fine goose pimples; minute muscle twitching, fine tremors; delicate body.
Mobile (*chala*)	Fast walking and talking; doing many things at once; restless eyes, eyebrows, hands, and feet; unstable joints; many dreams; loves traveling but does not stay at one place; swinging moods, shaky faith, scattered mind.
Clear (*vishada*)	Clairvoyant; understands immediately and forgets immediately; clear, empty mind; experiences void and loneliness.
Astringent (*kshaya*)	Dry choking sensation in the throat; hiccough, burping; loves oily foods and mushy soups; craves sweet, sour, and salty tastes; tendency toward constipation.

Pitta Dosha

Principally made up of fire and water, *pitta* expresses itself as the body's metabolic system. It governs digestion, absorption, assimilation, nutrition, color and complexion of skin, as well as body temperature. As with all *doshas*, *pitta* is present everywhere in the body, but its main site is the small intestine and it also concentrates in other areas including the eyes, skin, brain, and organs like the stomach, liver, gallbladder, and spleen. It is present in the gastric fire, bile, enzymes, and amino acids. It is also responsible for regulating body temperature and promoting hunger and thirst.

All that is received must undergo some process of digestion, including our thoughts, and *pitta* is mainly in charge of the digestion and assimilation of everything that goes into our body, from physical food and nutrients to sensory input. Its presence in neurotransmitters and neuropeptides plays a key role in the thinking process. *Pitta* helps to understand and transform information into knowledge and knowledge into wisdom.

Healthy *pitta* is associated with understanding, determination, courage, bravery, visual perception, and intelligence. Out of balance, it arouses anger, hatred, and jealousy, and gives rise to a wide variety of heat related and inflammatory disorders such as acid indigestion, gastritis, peptic ulcers, colitis, Crohn's disease, infections, rashes, migraines, and acne.

Characteristics of *Pitta*

Pitta individuals are of medium height and moderate in weight. They tend to have shapely bodies and good muscle tone. Their skin is warm with a coppery, fair, or reddish complexion, and can even appear to be yellowish. They may have some freckles and moles that tend to be reddish brown or blue in color. Their hair is silky, soft, light brown, blond, or red, with the tendency towards premature graying or baldness. Their eyes are penetrating and may be green, grayish blue, coppery, or yellow. Their chin and nose are also sharp and at times the nose can have a reddish tip.

Physiologically, *pitta* types have strong appetites and good digestion and metabolism. They often demand more food and generally have a powerful thirst, especially for cold drinks. Their body temperature is slightly high, they perspire easily, and their hands and feet are warm to the touch. They do not tolerate hot weather or over exposure to the sunlight and tend to sunburn easily.

Mentally, *pitta* types are bright and intelligent, and comprehend things easily and quickly. Emotionally, they have a tendency toward irritability, anger, jealousy, and even hatred. They are highly driven, natural born leaders, and often successful in what they set out to accomplish, although they can be perfectionists and dread failure, and be too hard on themselves as a result.

The qualities of *pitta* are hot, sharp, light, oily, liquid, sour, bitter, pungent, foul, spreading, and penetrating. These qualities and other features are revealed in the body of the *pitta* person, as shown in the chart of *pitta* attributes below.

Qualities in the *Pitta* Individual

Attributes	Constitutional Manifestations
Hot (*ushna*)	Good digestive fire; strong appetite; body temperature tends to be higher than average; hates heat; tendency toward gray hair with receding hairline or baldness; soft brown hair on the body and face.
Sharp (*tikshna*)	Sharp teeth, distinct eyes, pointed nose, tapering chin, heart-shaped face; good absorption and digestion; sharp memory and understanding; irritable; probing mind.
Light (*laghu*)	Light/medium body frame; does not tolerate bright light; fair shiny skin, bright eyes.
Oily (*snigdha*)	Soft oily skin, hair, and feces; sensitive to deep-fried food (which may cause headaches).
Liquid (*drava*)	Loose liquid stools; soft delicate muscles; excess urine, sweat, and thirst.
Sour (*amla*)	Sour acid stomach, acidic pH; sensitive teeth; excess salivation.
Bitter (*tikta*)	Bitter taste in the mouth; nausea; vomiting; repulsion toward bitter taste; cynical.
Pungent (*katu*)	Heartburn, burning sensations in general; strong feelings of anger and hate.
Foul smell (*visra*)	Fetid smell in mouth, soles of feet, and armpits.
Spreading (*saram*)	Rashes, hives, acne, inflammation all over the body or on certain areas; wants to spread his name and fame.

Attributes	Constitutional Manifestations
Red	Red flushed skin, eyes, cheeks, and nose; red color aggravates.
Yellow	Yellow eyes, skin, urine, and feces; jaundice; overproduction of bile; yellow color aggravates.

Kapha Dosha

Primarily made up of water and earth, *kapha* is the energy that forms all bodily structure and provides the cohesion that holds the cells together to give shape to organs and tissues. It also lubricates the joints, moisturizes the skin, and maintains *ojas* (vital essence and immunity). It gives strength to muscles and bones, protects the whole organism, promotes stability and memory retention, is in charge of bodily secretions, and is associated with emotions such as love, compassion, and forgiveness. When out of balance, it creates attachment, greed, and envy due to its heavy, static, slimy, and sticky qualities.

Excess *kapha* can cause low appetite, sluggish digestion, a feeling of heaviness, congestion, exhaustion, pallor, repeated colds, coughing, difficulty breathing, and excess sleep. It is also the primary factor in a variety of disorders, including diabetes, obesity, edema, congestive cardiac failure, hypertension, asthma, tumors, cysts, endometriosis, and fibrocystic changes.

Characteristics of *Kapha*

Kapha types have strong and well developed bodies. However, they also have a tendency to gain and retain excess weight. They often have good muscle development, a broad and expanded chest, and their joints, veins, and tendons are not prominent due to their well padded form. They have strong teeth and bones, their hair is thick, dark, soft, and wavy, and their skin is often hairy. They tend to have a fair complexion and their skin tends to be soft, moist, oily, and often cold and clammy to the touch. Their eyes are big and attractive, usually blue or black in color. Physiologically, they have a steady appetite and thirst, but they tend to have a slow digestion and metabolism.

Psychologically, they often have a great deal of love, compassion, patience, and forgiveness, but when out of balance they are more prone toward greed, attachment, possessiveness, and envy. They are not as quick to comprehend as *vata* and *pitta* types, but they have good memory retention.

Kapha has heavy, slow, cool, oily, liquid, smooth, dense, soft, static, sticky, viscous, cloudy, slimy, hard, and gross qualities. The manifestation of these qualities in the *kapha* constitution can be seen in the table of *kapha* attributes below.

Qualities in the *Kapha* Individual

Attributes	Constitutional Manifestations
Heavy (*guru*)	Heavy bones and muscles; large body frame; tends to be overweight; grounded; has a deep, heavy voice.
Slow (*manda*)	Walks and talks slowly; steady appetite with slow digestion and metabolism.
Cold (*shita*)	Cold clammy skin; repeated colds, congestion, and cough; desire for sweets and cold drinks.
Oily (*snigdha*)	Oily skin, hair, and feces; lubricated, unctuous joints and other organs.
Liquid (*drava*)	Congestive disorders; edema; excessive salivation; mucus.
Smooth (*shlakshna*)	Smooth skin; gentle, calm nature; smoothness of organs; gentle mind.
Dense (*sandra*)	Dense pad of fat; thick skin, hair, nails, and feces.
Soft (*mrudu*)	Soft pleasing look; love, care, compassion, kindness, and forgiveness.
Static (*sthira*)	Loves sitting, sleeping, and doing nothing.
Viscous	Slow, flowing movements; healthy, free moving joints; compact muscles, tissues, and organs; loves to hug; is deeply attached in love and relationships.
Cloudy (*vishada*)	Mind is cloudy and foggy in the morning; often desires coffee as a stimulant to start the day.
Slimy (*slakshna*)	Excess salivation; slow digestion; attachment.
Sweet (*madhu*)	Growth; fertility; increasing quantity of semen; craving for sweets.
Salty (*lavana*)	Tendency toward water retention; craving for salt.

Subtypes of the *Doshas*

Each of the *doshas* is divided into five subtypes that relate to various aspects of the body and govern its functions. One important aspect of Ayurvedic diagnosis is to determine which of the *doshic* subtypes are affected in any given case to narrow down and focus the treatment. When a *dosha* becomes imbalanced, its qualities can spread throughout the system and deposit themselves in any tissues, channels, and organs relating to the various *doshic* quadrants that have become predisposed or affected. Several doshic subtypes may be affected at the same time and often a specific treatment may address several subtypes simultaneously. Below is a list of the various doshic subtypes along with their related elements, locations, and functions, as well as signs and symptoms of imbalance and related disorders.

Subtypes of *Vata Dosha*

1. ***Prana Vayu*** (Inward and Downward Movement)

   Element: Ether/Space.

   Location: The center of the brain.

   Functions: Vital life force (*prana*); respiration, inhalation; sensory perception, flow of intelligence, memory, higher cerebral functions; movement of thoughts, feelings and emotions; intellect, ESP; swallowing, coughing, sneezing; pulsation and circulation along with *vyana vayu.*

   Signs and symptoms of imbalance: Hiccup, constant burping, palpitation, breathlessness, hoarseness, lack of concentration, anxiety, nervousness, fear, and anger.

   Disorders of *prana vayu*: Stroke paralysis, epilepsy, sleep apnea, Parkinson's disease, bronchitis, pneumonia, and asthma.

2. ***Udana Vayu*** (Upward Movement)

   Element: Air.

   Location: Diaphragm and throat.

   Functions: Stimulates speech, expression, effort, memory; upward movement of the diaphragm, exhalation; maintains skin color; carries spiritual energy upward.

   Signs and symptoms of imbalance: Depression, discoloration of the skin, hoarseness of voice, asthma, emphysema, memory loss, and speech disorders.

   Disorders of *udana vayu*: Ear, nose and throat diseases.

3. ***Samana Vayu*** (Balancing and Linear Movement)

Element: Fire.

Location: Abdominal viscera (mainly in the lower third of the stomach and small intestine).

Functions: Digestion, assimilation and absorption; secretes digestive juices, kindles the appetite; discrimination of essential and non-essential foodstuff; carries food through the intestines to the cecum; peristalsis.

Signs and symptoms of imbalance: Loss of appetite, indigestion, increase or decrease of peristalsis, nausea, intestinal pain, diarrhea, constipation, bloating, and lack of absorption and assimilation.

Disorders of *samana vayu*: Digestive disorders.

4. ***Vyana Vayu*** (Vehicle of Circulation)

Element: Water.

Location: Situated in the heart, moves throughout the entire body.

Functions: Maintains cardiac activity; arterial, venous and lymphatic circulation; nutrition, oxygenation; movement of joints and muscles, and reflex movement.

Signs and symptoms of imbalance: Poor circulation, ischemia (sudden lack of circulation), profuse sweating, sweating of the hands and feet, lack of oxygenation, edema, and muscle twitching.

Disorders of *vyana vayu*: Heart disease, hypertension, hypotension, and stroke.

5. ***Apana Vayu*** (Downward and Outward Movement)

Element: Earth.

Location: Colon, pelvic cavity and urinary tract.

Functions: Elimination of feces, gas, urine, sweat, menstrual blood, birthing of the fetus; sex urge, ovulation; nourishes the fetus during pregnancy; promotes conception (joining of sperm and ovum).

Signs and symptoms of imbalance: Constipation, diarrhea, retention of urine, frequent urination, profuse or absent menstruation, pain during menstruation, pain during ovulation, pain during sex, low backache, low sexual energy, premature ejaculation or orgasm, hemorrhoids and fissures.

Disorders of *apana vayu*: Diseases of the anus, colon, bladder, testicles, uterus, urinary tract, and miscarriage.

Subtypes of *Pitta Dosha*

1. *Pachaka Pitta* (Digestion)

   Element: Fire.

   Location: Upper GI tract.

   Functions: *Jathara agni* (digestive fire in stomach), digestion, absorption, assimilation of food; transformation of nutrients; includes hydrochloric acid, digestive enzymes, and pepsin.

   Signs and symptoms of imbalance: Hyperacidity, hypoglycemia, burning sensation in stomach, sugar cravings, and indigestion.

   Disorders of *pachaka pitta*: Gastritis, peptic ulcer, gastric reflux, and anorexia.

2. *Ranjaka Pitta* (Coloration, Formation of Blood Cells)

   Element: Water.

   Location: Liver and spleen, *bhuta agni* (digestive fire in the liver), stomach, pancreas, small intestine, and blood.

   Functions: Present as bile, gastric intrinsic factors, enzymes in the bone marrow and blood; gives color to the blood and all other tissues; synthesizes hemoglobin; metabolizes the five elements; produces white blood cells in the spleen.

   Signs and symptoms of imbalance: Liver, spleen and stomach dysfunction, anger, hatred, sensitivity to light, high cholesterol, and fatty diarrhea.

   Disorders of *ranjaka pitta*: Hepatitis, jaundice, gallstones, anemia, chronic fatigue syndrome, mononucleosis, fatty degenerative changes in the liver, gallstones.

3. *Sadhaka Pitta* (Comprehension)

   Element: Ether/Space.

   Location: Brain, heart, and heart chakra.

   Functions: Digests information; governs the mind, ego, intellect, and self-esteem; processes thoughts, feelings, and emotions; promotes awareness and comprehension.

   Signs and symptoms of imbalance: Lack of understanding and concentration, low self-esteem, misconceptions, anxiety, sadness, confusion, delusion, lack of direction and clarity, and hallucinations.

   Disorders of *sadhaka pitta*: Mental and emotional disorders, learning difficulty, insanity, neurological disorder.

4. *Alochaka Pitta* (Vision)

Element: Air.

Location: The eyes.

Functions: Optical perception, meaningful vision; maintains color and luster of the eyes.

Signs and symptoms of imbalance: Poor eyesight, far or short-sightedness, increased intraocular pressure, burning and redness of the eyes, styes, floaters, sensitivity to light.

Disorders of *alochaka pitta*: Glaucoma, cataracts (pitta/kapha), conjunctivitis, blepharitis, diminished vision.

5. *Bhrajaka Pitta* (Temperature)

Element: Earth.

Location: The skin.

Functions: Keeps skin warm; maintains normal tone, complexion and luster of the skin; absorbs medicines applied to skin; vitamin D absorption; tactile sense of touch.

Signs and symptoms of imbalance: Urticaria, hives, eczema, psoriasis, dermatitis, acne, anesthesia, tingling, numbness, and leukoderma

Disorders of *bhrajaka pitta*: Skin diseases.

Subtypes of *Kapha Dosha*

1. *Kledaka Kapha* (Liquefaction/Emulsification)

Element: Fire.

Location: Stomach and GI tract.

Functions: Present as the gastric mucous membrane (for protection from *pitta*); provides fluid for gastric secretions and hormones; digestion, emulsification/liquefaction of food; absorption, nourishment of *rasa dhatu* (plasma); hydration of cells and tissues; brings contentment after eating; provides confidence and courage.

Signs and symptoms of imbalance: Heaviness after meals, stomachache, indigestion, attachment and greed, nausea and vomiting (if *kledaka* is diminished).

Disorders of *kledaka kapha*: Anorexia, dyspepsia, peptic ulcer, hypochlorhydria, stomach tumor, gastritis, and peptic ulcer (if diminished).

2. *Avalambaka Kapha* (Respiration)

Element: Air.

Location: Chest and lungs (respiratory and cardiovascular systems).

Functions: Gaseous exchange; carries *prana*; supports all *kapha* systems in the body; protects and maintains tone of the lungs and heart; holds emotions, love, support, and compassion.

Signs and symptoms of imbalance: Respiratory congestion; laziness, grief and sadness in the lungs.

Disorders of *avalambaka kapha*: Lung disorders including bronchitis, bronchiectasis, asthma, pneumonia, emphysema, and tuberculosis.

3. *Bodhaka Kapha* (Taste Perception)

Element: Water.

Location: Oral cavity.

Functions: Taste perception, salivary glands, secretions; digestion (proteins, starches and carbohydrates); healing tissues; moistening of the throat and vocal cords.

Signs and symptoms of imbalance: Lack of or excess salivation, food cravings, sensitivity to sugar and carbohydrates, loss of taste, drooling, and thick, sticky saliva (may indicate dehydration or diabetes).

Disorders of *bodhaka kapha*: Bacterial infections of the mouth, gum infections, dental plaque, septic tonsillitis.

4. *Tarpaka Kapha* (Nourishment, Retention)

Element: Ether.

Location: The white matter of the brain.

Functions: Nourishes and protects the brain, senses and nerve cells; insulates nerves; cellular memory; present as cerebral spinal fluid; nourishes DNA molecules; lubricates the sinuses and nasal cavities.

Signs and symptoms of imbalance: Increased intracranial pressure, dizziness, sinus congestion, preoccupation, confusion, dullness of the senses, and mental fatigue.

Disorders of *tarpaka kapha*: Stroke paralysis, Parkinson's disease, brain tumors.

5. *Shleshaka Kapha* (Joint Movement)

Element: Earth.

Location: Joint spaces.

Functions: Present as sinovial fluid; lubricates joints; nourishes bones and periosteum, prevents bone decay, and promotes freedom of movement and emotions.

Signs and symptoms of imbalance: Cracking and popping joints, joint pain, stiffness, and swelling.

Disorders of *shleshaka kapha*: Osteoarthritis and rheumatoid arthritis.

Agni, the Fire of Digestion and Transformation

All that is taken in—be it food, herbs, or sensory perceptions—must be transformed by *agni*, or the fire principle. The concept of *agni* is deeply rooted in Vedic culture and exists on the microcosmic and macrocosmic levels. It is not only the fire of digestion, it is also the *yajna* or sacrificial fire. In the Vedic fire ceremony, it represents the mouth of God into which our negative tendencies and actions, symbolized by grains and seeds, are offered to purify ourselves on the subtle and causal levels. Internally, it represents our sacrifice of selfish interests into the fire of pure awareness. It is the great mediator and messenger between our lower and higher selves, and between the Earth and the atmospheric and celestial realms. It is the fire of the sun as well as the flame that blazes in the hearts and minds of all living things.

From an Ayurvedic perspective, *agni* is contained within *pitta dosha* and is present everywhere in the body, governing all metabolic activities. One of the primary sites of *agni* is the stomach. It is present there as *jathara agni* and governs the initial phase of digestion. Digestive secretions such as enzymes and hydrochloric acid are considered its fuel.

Agni is also present within each of the seven bodily tissues as *dhatu agni* and is in charge of the metabolic transformations of each tissue element. When *agni* is strong, food is digested properly and made available to every cell of the body. When *agni* becomes disturbed by factors such as *doshic* imbalance, improper diet and lifestyle, incompatible food combinations, and emotional factors, food does not get properly digested. This in turn leads to the formation of toxins in the GI tract. These toxins then get absorbed into the blood and spread throughout the body, accumulating and clogging the tissues, channels, and organs, as well as any weak or defective (predisposed) area (known as *khavaigunya*).

There are forty main types of *agni* present in the body that relate to the five elements, *doshic* subtypes, organs, tissues, waste products, and cellular metabolism. In order to maintain overall health it is essential that the various components of *agni* be balanced. First and foremost, the best support for keeping *agni* strong and healthy is proper self-care through diet and lifestyle. Our ability to digest food or herbs properly is the result of a balanced *agni*. Even herbs and supplements can cause *ama* when the organism is not able to digest and absorb them.

Furthermore, to detoxify the body we must burn *ama*. For this reason, Ayurveda places great emphasis on kindling *agni* even when following a deep detoxification programs such as *Panchakarma*, during which easily digestible food is given to keep the *agni* burning bright. Fasting from food or drink over prolonged periods is not recommended, as this approach can eventually weaken the digestive fire and cause toxins to stagnate in the body, putting stress upon the tissues, organs, and channels. In this sense, excess fasting can create a sort of toxic traffic jam that can lead to what is often referred to as a healing crisis.

There are four clinical varieties of *agni* that can be recognized through Ayurvedic assessment: *Sama agni, vishama agni, tikshna agni*, and *manda agni*. These are specific states of the digestive fire as they relate to the *doshas*.

Sama agni is balanced or *tridoshic*. A person with *sama agni* can eat a wide variety of foods without any disturbance of the digestion, absorption, or elimination. This type of person has a strong constitution and good immunity.

Vishama agni, which is variable metabolism, is often associated with *vata dosha*. Here the appetite and digestion are irregular, and almost any kind of food can cause gas, bloating, indigestion, and constipation. If left unchecked, it can also lead to further *vata* disorders.

Tikshna agni relates to *pitta dosha*. In this case, the hot, sharp qualities of *pitta* create a hyper-metabolic condition that is characterized by an intense appetite, dry mouth, acid indigestion, heartburn, hypoglycemia, and eventually gastrointestinal inflammation and ulcers.

Manda agni relates to *kapha dosha*. It is slow and dull, and causes hypo-metabolism. People with this kind of *agni* gain weight easily and often feel heaviness in the stomach after eating. This kind of *agni* can cause diminished appetite, lethargy, obesity, edema, congestion, allergies, and a wide variety of *kapha* disorders.

There is also a specialized *agni* related to the *sadhaka pitta* present in the grey matter of the brain and the heart chakra that is responsible for proper understanding, comprehension, and the sense of I am-ness. It governs the transformation of sensation into thoughts, feelings, and emotions, and that of knowledge into wisdom.

When *agni* is balanced, the individual enjoys vitality, a bright complexion, vigor, enthusiasm, mental clarity, a positive outlook, a clean tongue, and good digestion and elimination. If *agni* is impaired, then it can cause confusion, fatigue, exhaustion, foul breath, constipation, diarrhea, poor digestion, and a thick coating on the tongue.

Dhatus: Seven Bodily Tissues

Ayurveda views that the body is composed of seven *dhatus*, or basic tissue elements. These are: *Rasa* (plasma), *rakta* (blood), *mamsa* (muscle), *meda* (adipose tissue), *asthi* (bone), *majja* (marrow and nerve), and *shukra/artava* (male and female reproductive tissues). Each of the seven tissues is formed in stages and takes 5 days to be developed from an unripe stage to a mature stage. So it takes 35 days for all the bodily tissues to complete a full cycle of nourishment. Food is transformed into plasma from the basic nutrient precursors in the digestive tract. This plasma nourishes the blood, which in turn flows on to provide nourishment to the muscle, fat, marrow, nerve, and reproductive tissues with the help of the various *agni* components within each of the tissues.

The ancient texts describe three basic processes in which each of the tissues receives its nourishment. The first process is that of irrigation, by which nutrients are carried through the general circulation to nourish the tissues. The second is selectivity, by which each tissue, through its inherent intelligence, selects what it needs from the stream of nutrients provided. And the third is transformation, by which the unstable or unripe tissue is transformed into a stable or mature tissue through the power of *agni*.

Each of the *dhatus* has a superior byproduct (*upadhatu*) as well as an inferior byproduct or waste product (*mala*). The health of the seven tissues can be inferred by the proper formation and quality of these byproducts. Below is a basic list of the seven *dhatus*, their functions, and associated *doshas*, followed by a brief description of each tissue element.

Dhatus	**Functions**	**Associated *Doshas***
Rasa: Plasma (lymphatic system, serum, white blood cells)	Nutrition	*Kapha*
Rakta: Blood (red blood cells)	Life giving energy	*Pitta*
Mamsa: Muscle	Plastering, shaping	*Kapha*
Meda: Adipose tissue / fat	Lubrication	*Kapha*
Asthi: Bone	Support, protection	*Vata*
Majja: Marrow, nerve tissue, and connective tissue	To fill spaces	*Kapha*
Shukra: Male reproductive tissue	Procreation	*Kapha / Pitta*
Artava: Female reproductive tissue	Procreation	*Pitta / Kapha*

Rasa (Plasma)

Rasa is the plasma portion of the blood. It is associated with the lymphatic system and includes the lymph and white blood cells. Its unique function is *prinana*, which literally means "nourishment." Because it is the first tissue to be formed, it provides the foundation for the rest of the tissues. Healthy *rasa* is associated with smooth, soft skin, clear perception, faith, and love. The byproduct or *upadhatu* of *rasa* is the topmost layer of the skin, lactation, and menstruation; its waste product or *mala* is the precursor of *kapha dosha*.

Rakta (Blood)

Rakta is the red blood cells, which provide *jivana*, or the life supporting energy to the body. *Rakta* helps to carry *prana*, oxygen, and nutrients from the lungs and the GI tract to the entire system. It also carries out waste products to the lungs in the form of carbon dioxide and other wastes to the organs of elimination. A healthy *rakta dhatu* promotes energy, vitality, warmth, a vibrant complexion, lustrous eyes, red lips, rosy cheeks, and a pinkish color of the nail beads, soles, and palms. Optimal function of *rakta* also promotes intelligence. Its *upadhatu* is the blood vessels, granulation tissue, small tendons, and sinews; its *mala* is the precursor of *pitta dosha*.

Mamsa (Muscle)

Mamsa is the muscle tissue and is derived mainly from *kapha dosha*. It performs the function of *lepana*, or plastering, provides the body with shape and movement, and the person with the ability to express emotions and thoughts through bodily movement. Proper formation of this tissue gives power both mentally and physically, and is associated with courage, high self-esteem, and ambition, as well as a loving, compassionate, and forgiving nature. Optimal *mamsa dhatu* promotes good muscle tone and development, stability, and frankness. Its *upadhatu* is the other six layers of skin and subcutaneous fat; its *mala* is exuded from the body's orifices as earwax, nasal crust, sebaceous secretions, tooth tartar, and smegma.

Meda (Adipose or Fat)

Meda is the adipose tissue and includes all loose connective tissues, fat, phospholipids, cholesterol, and other lipids. One of the main functions of *meda dhatu* is to provide lubrication (*snehana*) to the joints, organs, and tissues. Fat tissue provides protection as well as insulation to keep the body warm. Fats are essential for the formation of cells and to supply the energy needed for all cellular activity. Healthy *meda* gives beauty to the eyes and hair, softness and shine to the skin, flexibility to the joints, strength to teeth and nails, and promotes a deep, melodious voice. Its *upadhatu* is tendons, sinews, and flat muscles; its *mala* is sweat.

Asthi (Bone)

The bone tissue is primarily composed of the earth element and provides *dharana*, or support. It also gives shape and protects vital organs. Along with the help of the muscle tissue, it enables self-expression through movement. When *asthi dhatu* is properly nourished, it provides strong bones, joints, teeth, hair, and nails. Optimal bone development gives strength, stability, firm determination, and healthy personal boundaries. Its *upadhatu* is teeth and cartilage; its *mala* is hair and nails.

Majja (Bone Marrow and Nerve)

Majja has the function of *purana*, or filling of spaces, with knowledge, fluids, or information. It includes the red and yellow bone marrow, as well as the brain and spinal cord. The filling of the hollow spaces of the bones helps to prevent the accumulation of excess *vata*, which already has an affinity to the bone tissue. *Majja* carries sensory and motor impulses and is the vehicle for the intellect and the communication between the various cells, organs, and systems of the body. Psychologically speaking, it fills us with the sense of who we are as individuals. *Majja* is made up mainly of *kapha*. Healthy *majja* imparts well lubricated skin, a melodious voice, big beautiful eyes, and strong joints, as well as general strength, intelligence, the desire to learn, and a humorous, loving, and affectionate nature. Its *upadhatu* is lacrimal secretions; its *mala* is the oily secretions in the eyes.

Shukra /*Artava* (Male and Female Reproductive Tissues)

The last tissue to be nourished is the reproductive tissue. In Sanskrit, sperm is referred to as *shukra*. It is cool in nature and has *kapha* like qualities. *Artava* is the ovum, or the female egg. It is hot with *pitta* attributes. A woman's orgasmic fluids are referred to as female *shukra*. The function of these tissues is *prajanana*, which means "procreation." They provide sexual energy and emotional release. The refined essence that forms from *shukra* and *artava* is *ojas*, the life giving reserve of the body. Signs of robust *shukra* are an attractive body, lustrous eyes, well formed sexual organs, healthy hair, teeth, and skin, good immunity, happiness, creativity, and a strong but balanced sexual energy. The *upadhatu* of these tissues is *ojas*; their *mala* are the secretions at the time of ejaculation and orgasm.

Ojas (The Pure Essence of All Bodily Tissues)

Once all of the tissue elements have been formed, the end product is *ojas*, which is the pure essence of all the tissues. *Ojas* is the life giving sap that maintains strength, vigor, and vitality. Each tissue forms its own *ojas* to some degree, but it is mainly formed as the superior byproduct of the reproductive tissue. It is present in all hormonal secretions and is the prime substance involved in the support of the immune system. *Ojas* is also the essential fuel for stabilizing and concentrating the mind upon a spiritual aim, and is vital for the practice of meditation. For this reason, the ancient *rishis* encouraged the conservation of vital essence through a disciplined diet and lifestyle.

Herbs and the Tissues

In Ayurvedic herbology, herbs are categorized according to the tissues they affect. For example, many alterative herbs have a bitter taste and affect the plasma and blood, and also reduce the adipose tissue. Nutritive tonics and rejuvenating herbs like *shatavari* and *ashwagandha* nourish the muscle, fat, and reproductive tissues. Many warming and stimulating spices like ginger, black pepper, and *pippali* improve metabolism and are helpful for maintaining a healthy balance of the fat tissue. So a single herb can have an effect on a number of tissues. Therefore, herbs should be selected carefully so as to keep formulas simple yet dynamic. Let's say someone has a condition such as hepatitis C and also suffers from *pitta* types of emotional disturbances such as anger and irritability. In this case, herbs like *bhringaraj* and *brahmi* (gotu kola), both of which have alterative and nervine properties, could be used to address the underlying *pitta* condition by clearing excess heat from the plasma and blood, as well as cooling the nerves and calming the mind.

Below is a simplified list of the seven bodily tissues and examples of herbal properties that have specific effects on them.

Rasa: Alteratives, nutritive tonics, demulcents, stimulants, and diaphoretics.

Rakta: Blood tonics, alteratives, and purgatives.

Mamsa: Nutritive and rejuvenating tonics, and alteratives.

Meda: Bitter tonics, alteratives, stimulants, decongestants, expectorants, and diuretics.

Asthi: Nutritive and rejuvenating tonics, and carminatives.

Majja: Nervine tonics and sedatives.

Shukra/Artava: Rejuvenating and nutritive tonics, aphrodisiacs, and emmenagogues.

If there is disorder of the *doshas*, the bodily tissues will be directly affected. So, in the assessment of disease, it is important to understand which of the *doshas* are involved and which of the tissues they are affecting. For example, if *vata* is increased and is affecting the bone tissue, it can cause too much space, which may lead to osteoporosis. If *pitta*, which is hot, sharp, and spreading, affects the blood, it can create hives, acne, and rashes like psoriasis or eczema. When there is excess *kapha* it can cause an over production of fat tissue, leading to obesity. Conversely, if *vata* is affecting the fat tissue, it can cause emaciation.

Agni and the Tissues

Each tissue element has its own digestive fire or *dhatu agni*, which helps it to cook and refine the essence of the preceding tissue. If the digestive ability of the tissue is diminished, there will be an accumulation of that unprocessed tissue, which can lead to conditions of increase or excess (*dhatu vruddhi*). If the *agni* of a tissue is too strong it burns the nutrients, which can lead to conditions of decrease or deficiency (*dhatu kshaya*). Generally speaking, if there is low *agni* in the fat tissue there will be too much fat in the body (*meda vruddhi*); if there is too much *agni* there will be an under production of fat (*meda kshaya*) caused by over cooking, and therefore the person will have difficulty gaining weight. Similarly, excess bone tissue (*asthi vruddhi*) can cause bone spurs or micro calcification, whereas too little (*asthi kshaya*) can create hair loss, degenerative forms of arthritis, or osteoporosis.

If we understand not only which tissue is affected but also how it is affected, this can further guide us in choosing the proper course of herbal treatment. In an increased tissue, bitter, pungent, astringent, and stimulating herbs are helpful because they have a reducing action. If there is deficient tissue, then nutritive and rejuvenating tonics are best. For example, if there is deficient blood, then blood building tonics such as *amalaki, haritaki*, or nettles can be given; and if there is tissue excess, then lighter and more purifying herbs like dandelion, burdock, or *neem* can be used. An increase in the plasma tissue, which is watery and *kapha* in nature, can lead to congestive disorders. In this case, warming and stimulating herbs like ginger or cinnamon can help. If there is a decrease in plasma, then there can be dehydration, weight loss, etc., so moistening and nourishing herbs like licorice and *shatavari* can be chosen to replenish the water element in the body.

Srotamsi: Bodily Channels and Systems

There are many channels or systems in the human body known as *srotamsi* (the plural for *srotas*, which means "channel"). These are the pathways through which all substances and energies are circulated in the body. Each *srotas* is responsible for maintaining specific functions such as digestion, absorption, and assimilation, as well as circulation, respiration, elimination, and so on. *Dhatu srotamsi* (channels supplying the tissue layers) are structural, while *mala srotamsi* (waste channels) are more functional in nature.

Each *srotas* is made up of a *mula* (root), a *marga* (passageway) and a *mukha* (mouth or opening). Many of these channels, which have clearly defined pathways, relate closely to the systems of Western physiology. A good example of this is *annavaha srotas*, or the channel of food, which relates to the upper GI tract. Its *mula* is the esophagus and fundus of the stomach, and its *marga* is the GI tract up to the ileocecal valve, which is its *mukha*.

When the channels are functioning properly, all of the *dhatus* receive the required nourishment and the body expels its wastes efficiently. If this flow is hindered by the vitiation of the *doshas* or by the accumulation of toxins, disease can manifest.

Ayurveda recognizes four main types of imbalances related to the *srotamsi* and known as *sroto dushti*:

1. ***Atipravrutti***: When there is excess or overflow, as in diarrhea or vomiting.

2. ***Sanga***: When there is stagnation of flow due to an accumulation of toxins, bodily wastes, or excess tissues, as in the case of constipation, blood clots, arteriosclerosis, and lymphatic congestion.

3. ***Sira granthi***: When there is dilution, growth, or swelling, as in the case of tumors or diverticulosis.

4. ***Vimarga gamanam***: When the flow goes in the wrong direction and even out of the wrong channels, as in bleeding of the nose, lungs or gums, pleurisy, hematoma, fistula, or perforation.

There may also be more than one of these conditions happening simultaneously, or one condition may lead into another. For example, hemorrhoids can be viewed as a combination of stagnation and swelling, which in time can cause a hemorrhoid to rupture and create a false passage and bleeding.

From an Ayurvedic perspective, there are 16 major channels in the body. I have classified these *srotamsi* below according to their main functions and how they relate to the Western model of physiology, as well as to the causes and some of the main signs and symptoms of *sroto dushti*, or imbalance.

1. ***Pranavaha srotas*:** The channel carrying the breath and vital energy, which relates to the respiratory system and the *maha srotas* (entire GI tract).

Causes of *sroto dushti*: Inhalation of dust and debris, pollution, suppression of natural urges, and excess intake of dry foods.

Signs and symptoms: Colds, cough, congestion, difficulty breathing, wheezing, hoarseness, and asthma.

2. ***Annavaha srotas*:** The channel carrying food, which relates to the digestive system.

Causes of *sroto dushti*: Untimely eating, over or under eating, poor food combining, eating while upset, traveling, and excessive intake of fluids.

Signs and symptoms: Anorexia, indigestion, nausea, vomiting, and diarrhea.

3. ***Udaka/Ambuvaha srotas*:** The channel carrying water and governing water metabolism, which is an aspect of the digestive system.

Causes of *sroto dushti*: Excess consumption of salty, sweet, or sour tastes, profuse sweating, excess consumption of alcohol, over exercise, excess *ama* clogging the pores of the skin, over hunger or thirst.

Signs and symptoms: Dry throat, lips, tongue, and palate; skin remains tented after being pinched, excess thirst, dehydration, extreme debility, and edema.

4. ***Rasavaha srotas*:** The channel carrying plasma and lymph, which relates to the lymphatic system and to some aspects of the circulatory system.

Causes of *sroto dushti*: Excess alcohol or hot spicy foods, or cold, dry food, summer season, anger, criticism, too much fluid intake.

Signs and symptoms: Anorexia, malaise and fatigue, lack of luster, lack of faith, low self-esteem, nausea, rashes, fainting, anemia, impotency, repeated colds and flu, and heaviness in the heart region.

5. ***Raktavaha srotas*:** The channel carrying the hemoglobin portion of the blood, which is also an aspect of the circulatory system.

Causes of *sroto dushti*: Hot spicy, fermented, or salty foods, smoking marijuana or tobacco, and over exposure to the sun.

Signs and symptoms: Skin diseases, burning sensations, infections, bleeding disorders, jaundice, burning hemorrhoids, and a wide variety of inflammatory diseases.

6. ***Mamsavaha srotas*:** The channel carrying nutrients to the muscle tissue, which relates to the muscular system.

Causes of *sroto dushti*: Sleeping immediately after eating, excess intake of heavy foods like cheese, milk, meats, or yogurt; overeating, improper exercise (too much or not enough), trauma, improper posture, and liver diseases.

Signs and symptoms: Muscle strains and pains, tics, spasms, excess earwax and nasal crust, myoma, boils, and goiter.

7. ***Medavaha srotas*:** The channel carrying nutrients to the fat tissue, which relates to the adipose system.

Causes of *sroto dushti*: Sedentary life, sleeping in the daytime, slow metabolism, excess intake of heavy, rich, and fatty foods.

Signs and symptoms: Profuse sweating, obesity, pre-diabetic conditions, excess thirst, and lethargy after meals.

8. ***Asthivaha srotas*:** The channel carrying nutrients to the bone tissue, which relates to the skeletal system.

Causes of *sroto dushti*: Traumatic injury, *vata* provoking foods, poor absorption, mineral depletion, muscle tension, excessive wear and tear, sedentary lifestyle, and genetic factors.

Signs and symptoms: White spots or cracking of the nails, cracking of the teeth, hair loss (nails, hair, and teeth are closely associated with *asthi dhatu*), bone loss, cracking and popping of the joints, and T.M.J. bone pain.

9. *Majjavaha srotas*: The channel carrying nutrients to the bone marrow, which relates to the nervous system.

Causes of *sroto dushti*: *Vata* provoking foods, poor food combining, trauma to the bone such as crushing or cerebral injury, over stimulation, exposure to radiation, heavy metal toxicity.

Signs and symptoms: Lack of coordination, joint pains, giddiness, fainting, tingling, numbness, internal burning sensation, and loss of speech or memory.

10. *Shukravaha srotas*: The channel governing the male reproductive system.

Causes of *sroto dushti*: Emotional upset, poor nutrition, trauma to the scrotum, venereal diseases, too much sex, very hot baths, tight underwear, suppression of sexual fluids, and steroid hormones.

Signs and symptoms: Impotency, low libido, premature or painful ejaculation, low back pain, and prostatitis.

11. *Artavavaha srotas*: The channel governing the female reproductive system.

Causes of *sroto dushti*: Excessive douching, emotional upset, venereal diseases, too much sex, birth control medications, steroid hormones, improper lifestyle during pregnancy, and genetic predisposition.

Signs and symptoms: All disorders of the female reproductive system, low libido, low back pain, vaginal infections, all menstrual disorders, and pain during sex.

12. *Mutravaha srotas*: The channel carrying urine, which relates to the urinary system.

Causes of *sroto dushti*: Suppression of urination, urinating too frequently (without urge), insufficient water intake, excess consumption of nightshades, and eating too much hot spicy foods.

Signs and symptoms: Excess or scanty urination, dehydration, high blood pressure, uremia, chronic constipation, profuse sweating, urinary tract infection, incontinence, painful urination, kidney stones, and renal failure.

13. *Purishavaha srotas*: The channel carrying feces, which relates to the excretory system.

Causes of *sroto dushti*: Poor diet, incompatible food combining, suppression of the urge to defecate, straining during bowel movement, excessive eating or snacking, weak digestive fire, food poisoning, and fermented foods.

Signs and symptoms: Constipation, excessive bowel movements, bloating, dry stools, diarrhea, indigestion, malabsorption, fissures, hemorrhoids, fistula, diverticulosis, parasites, and bacterial infections.

14. *Svedavaha srotas*: The channel carrying sweat, which relates to the sebaceous system.

Causes of *sroto dushti*: Extremely hot, dry or cold climates, over exposure to the sun or heat, excessive exercise, emotional imbalances, excess intake of salt, yogurt, sugar, and hot spicy foods.

Signs and symptoms: Over or under perspiration, roughness of the skin, burning sensations of the skin, horripilation, acne, and any skin condition.

15. *Stanyavaha srotas*: The channel carrying the nutrients for lactation, which is related to the female hormonal system.

Cause of *sroto dushti*: Poor food combining, improper diet, any factors that affect *rasa dhatu* (lactation is a byproduct of *rasa dhatu*), and *vata* imbalances.

Signs and symptoms: Scanty or absent flow of breast milk, yeast infection, mastitis, and tenderness.

16. *Manovaha srotas*: The channel of the mind, or psychological aspect, which is also connected to the yogic metaphysical anatomy, i.e., *chakras*, *nadis*, and *koshas*, or bodily sheaths.

Causes of *sroto dushti*: Intense grief, fear, anger, obstructed flow of prana, toxins, recreational drugs, planetary influences, identification with thoughts, feelings, and emotions, trauma, obsession, dysfunctions of the senses, *karmic* influences, and *samskaras* (latent tendencies in the mind).

Signs and symptoms: Confusion, delusion, insomnia, depression, lack of focus or concentration, restless mind, fixation on thoughts, forgetfulness, negative thoughts, compulsive behaviors, and all emotional and psychological imbalances.

A Holistic and Individualized Approach

Prakruti and Inner Harmony

Ayurveda is a system of medicine that has evolved from practical, philosophical, and spiritual insight. It is also an art of daily living and a science of self-understanding that empowers everyone to take control and responsibility for their own health and well being with its common-sense approach.

The Ayurvedic system believes that each person has a unique constitution, or *prakruti*—an individual combination of physical, mental, and emotional characteristics. This individual constitution is determined by the specific combination of *vata, pitta,* and *kapha* at the time of conception and birth, and is recorded as a genetic code that is expressed both physically (as disease proneness) and mentally (as behavior and emotional response). It is influenced by factors such as the genetics, diet, lifestyle, and physical and mental state of the parents around the time of conception.

Everyone has all three *doshas* in their *prakruti* to varying degrees, although one and sometimes two tend to be predominant while the others remain secondary. According to the classical texts, there are 7 constitutional types: *Vata*; *Pitta*; *Kapha*; *Vata-Pitta*; *Pitta-Kapha*; *Vata-Kapha*; and *Vata-Pitta-Kapha* (equal). There are innumerable variations of these 7 types of *prakruti*, depending upon the ratio of each *dosha* in the individual constitution. Of all types, the last one, with equal *Vata-Pitta-Kapha*, is the most rare. Some schools of thought differentiate between say, *vata-pitta* and *pitta-vata*, depending on which of the *doshas* is slightly higher in the dual *doshic* constitution. Others point out the specific ratios by numbering each *dosha* according to its predominance (for example, V3 P2 K1, and so on), or using percentages (such as V30% P50% K20%). In any case, the main point is to determine which of the *doshas* are the most predominant, so as to counteract their effects through diet and lifestyle, as well as appropriate herbal therapies.

Many factors, both internal and external, can disturb the balance of the *doshas* and bring about changes that can lead to imbalance and disease. Some of these factors include emotional and physical stress, improper food combinations and choices, seasonal and weather

Part II: The Ayurvedic Approach to Health

changes, physical trauma, and work and family relationships. These changes are referred to in Sanskrit as *vikruti.*

If we understand how these factors affect the individual on a constitutional level, we can discern the appropriate actions to nullify or minimize their effects and eliminate the causes of imbalance, preventing or counteracting the disease process. Within the body there is a constant interaction between the original nature (*prakruti*) and the deviation from it (*vikruti*). When we understand the cause of *vikruti,* we can work toward re-establishing the original balance of *prakruti.*

As a general rule, the predominant *dosha* of the constitution determines the individual proneness toward particular diseases and disorders. This is why understanding our own constitution is a valuable tool for maintaining health. *Vata* types will tend to experience more *vata* conditions, while *pitta* types will tend to suffer from *pitta* disorders, and *kapha* types from *kapha* imbalances. For example, *pitta* individuals have more hot, sharp, and oily qualities than any other *dosha.* Therefore, they are more likely to suffer from an increase in these qualities than the *vata* or *kapha* individuals, who tend be colder in nature.

Yet it should be understood that not only *vata* people experience *vata* disorders, nor do only *pitta* people have *pitta* imbalances, or only *kapha* people suffer from *kapha* diseases. If anyone is exposed long enough to a particular quality, be it hot, wet, dry, etc., the internal environment can develop signs and symptoms of an increase of that quality. For example, exposure to cold damp weather can cause a *kapha* condition like the common cold with congestion and cough, no matter what the individual constitution may be, if the external condition is strong enough.

A helpful consideration is that when a disease is caused by any of the secondary *doshas* in the constitution it can be easily cured, whereas it is more difficult to treat if it is caused by the predominant *dosha,* due to the strong presence of that *dosha* in the constitution. Clinically, it is vital to detect any imbalanced *doshas* and to understand all the causative factors involved, so as to remove them to whatever degree possible to support the body's healing process.

In a situation where the causative *dosha* is different from the predominant *dosha* in the original *prakruti,* emphasis may need to be placed upon that causative *dosha* before the attention can be shifted to a more constitutionally based treatment. For example, when *vata* is high it can aggravate *pitta,* causing inflammatory conditions, just as the wind can cause a fire to spread. Providing that *vata* is the main cause and the symptoms of *pitta* are mild, then treating *vata* can help to relieve the secondary *pitta* condition without any direct treatment to *pitta*.

Then again, if *pitta* is provoked to the point that it presents a danger to the overall health of the system, it should not be overlooked, as it needs to be treated first regardless of the causative *dosha*. In any case, when treating the branches of the tree, it is important not to lose sight of the roots. Furthermore, both states of the *doshas* (*prakruti* and *vikruti*) along the causative factors of a given situation should be considered when assessing a case. The aim should always be to revert the disease process back to the inner harmony of the individual constitution. In other words, to bring any *vikruti* back to the original *prakruti*.

Management of Dosha

One of the first steps in managing health from an Ayurvedic perspective lies in understanding the individual constitution and which *dosha(s)* may be out of balance. This is tremendously useful when selecting a specific herbal treatment. Ayurveda classifies herbs in relation to their taste, action, post-digestive effect, and qualities (heavy or light, dry or wet, and so on). Based on this energetic model, not only herbs but also foods, culinary spices, and daily healthy habits can be used to counter the qualities of any disturbed *dosha(s)*. For instance, if there is excessive dryness in the body due to increased *vata*, moistening herbs such as licorice or marshmallow root can be used, as well as adding healthy oils into the diet. If there is excess heat and inflammation related to *pitta dosha*, cooling herbs such as *neem* or coriander can be used, as well as integrating cooling foods like fresh cilantro or coconut into the diet. For accumulated dampness causing cough and congestion, warming decongestants can be used to reduce excess *kapha*.

Priority is first given to the most aggravated *dosha*, then to the secondary *dosha*. If the *doshas* are relatively balanced, emphasis can be placed on general management of the predominant *dosha(s)* in the individual constitution to maintain optimal health. Since seasonal factors can also have a negative influence on the overall health, general preventative measures should be taken, such as following *vata* pacifying guidelines during the fall and winter, managing *pitta* in the late spring and summer, and avoiding the increase of *kapha* in the winter and early spring. Below are some basic tips for managing each of the *doshas*.

Vata Management (*Vato Pakrama*)

Vata has cold, dry, light, mobile, subtle, and clear qualities. To manage *vata dosha* it is important to select herbs, foods, and therapies that have the opposite qualities (warm, moistening, heavy, and grounding). Warm oil massage and steam baths, as well as eating primarily cooked, unctuous, and nourishing foods are good examples of how to pacify *vata*. The three tastes that pacify *vata* are sweet, sour, and salty, all of which have heavy, nourishing, and moistening qualities.

Due to its mobile or erratic quality, developing a daily routine for meal times, exercise, sleeping, meditation, etc., is one of the best ways to stabilize and calm this *dosha*. Furthermore, *vata* individuals will respond much better to other forms of therapy, herbal and otherwise, once these calming routines are established. The use of sweet, heavy, and nutritive tonic herbs and foods is also beneficial, since *vata* types tend toward deficiency due to their cold, dry, and light nature, which can lead to depletion of bodily tissues (*dhatu kshaya*).

When *vata* is increased in the colon, its main site, it can cause bloating, gas, and abdominal discomfort. Here carminative herbs like fennel, ginger, or *ajwan* can be used to help dispel gas. Due to the tendency of *vata* toward constipation, laxative herbs are often needed, but it is crucial to make the appropriate choice for each individual case. Dry forms of constipation are best treated with moistening herbs like licorice, marshmallow, or ground flaxseed. as well as the traditional preparation *Gandarva haritaki*. Psyllium seed is also considered to be moistening, but should always be taken with plenty of water. In my experience, it can cause gas and further aggravate constipation in individuals with dryness in the colon. Adding more healthy oils and *ghee* into the diet and drinking plenty of water everyday can help to create more moisture as well.

In the case of chronic constipation with little to no elimination, using strong laxative herbs like cascara sagrada, rhubarb, or senna may be necessary for a short period of time. If there is an obstruction, *basti* (enema) therapy should be used first to help break down and clear the blockage. Once that is successfully achieved, it is best to gradually switch from a strong laxative to a moistening or bulking one. Treating chronic constipation can be an arduous process that requires patience and discipline, especially in regards to following an appropriate diet and lifestyle to support the herbal treatment.

To both prevent and treat constipation, the Ayurvedic compound *triphala* can be used. This compound is quite unique in that it is an effective laxative as well as a bowel tonic that helps to improve the tone of the colon and regulates normal peristalsis. (See *Triphala*.)

Vata types are prone to a variable appetite and digestion. Therefore, warm pungent herbs can help to kindle their digestive fire and promote the digestion, absorption, and assimilation of food. It should be noted that when taken in excess, pungent taste may increase *vata*, if the substance used has an excessively hot quality, such as cayenne. Salty taste helps to kindle the appetite and promote digestion, and it can also act as a mild laxative. In Ayurveda there are many compounds that combine various salts with hot, pungent, and carminative herbs like *hingwastak churna*, which are used to treat weak digestion and obstructive *vata* disorders of the GI tract.

Demulcent herbs, which are mainly heavy, soft, and sweet and are often classified as nutritive or rejuvenating tonics, are great for *vata*, since these herbs help to protect and moisten the mucous membranes and skin, and to nourish *rasa dhatu*. In other words, these herbs help to increase and maintain the water element in the organism and counteract the dry, light, and rough qualities of *vata*.

Nervines are also very important in the treatment of *vata* conditions. Some nervines have more tonic properties that improve the strength and function of the nervous system, which tends to get depleted due to the hyperactive nature of *vata*. Other nervines are more sedative and antispasmodic, and can help in the treatment of *vata* ailments such as muscle cramps, spasms, insomnia, and anxiety. Nourishing herbs like *ashwagandha* and *vidari* have both tonic and sedative properties. Herbs like *brahmi* or gotu kola, *shankapushpi*, *jatamansi*, or skullcap are considered to yield tonic, stimulating, and sedative properties, depending upon what the body requires at the time.

Pitta Management (*Pitta Pakrama*)

Pitta dosha has hot, sharp, oily, light, and spreading qualities. *Pitta* management therapies are mainly cooling and calming to the body and mind. A few basic lifestyle recommendations to manage *pitta* are: Avoiding over exposure to the sun, fermented foods and drinks, deep-fried or hot spicy foods, and excess salt intake. The three tastes that pacify *pitta* are bitter, sweet, and astringent, with bitter being the coldest of the three.

Alterative herbs, which are predominately bitter in taste and have a cold *virya* (energy), are often used to dispel heat caused by increased *pitta* in the liver and blood. For this reason, they help to treat fever and infection, as well as a variety of inflammatory *pitta* conditions.

Since *pitta* is also light and spreading, it responds well to nutritive tonic herbs, many of which have a sweet taste and heavy quality. Herbs possessing both sweet and bitter tastes like *shatavari*, wild yam, or *vidari* are true *pitta* tonics. Such herbs can be taken for long periods of time without depleting the body like many primarily bitter herbs tend to do.

Pitta types often have a strong or sharp digestive fire (*tikshna agni*) and are prone to acid indigestion, heartburn, and even gastrointestinal inflammation and ulcers. Here demulcent herbs, which are typically sweet and moistening, like licorice, slippery elm, and marshmallow root can help to cool, protect, and promote healing to the mucous membranes.

Diarrhea, which often accompanies conditions related to high *pitta* in the GI tract, can also be corrected with demulcent and astringent herbs. A perfect herb for this is psyllium seed. Being both sweet and astringent, it helps to absorb the hot and liquid qualities of *pitta*.

The main therapy in Ayurveda for treating excess *pitta* is purgation therapy, or *virechana karma*. This therapy helps to clear *pitta* from the small intestine, moving it downward and out of the body. *Virechana karma* also regulates normal liver and gallbladder function. Purgation is also useful for *pitta* forms of constipation caused by dryness due to excess heat. Here cooling purgatives like rhubarb, senna, *trivrit*, or aloe vera (*kumari*) juice can be used along with demulcent herbs to provide moisture and lubrication. Purgation therapy is best employed by a skilled practitioner and is most successful when the body is first prepared for it, as when it is part of a *Panchakarma* (deep cleansing and rejuvenating) program and the excess *ama* (toxins) and *dosha* have been coaxed out of the deeper tissues into the GI tract.

Another major form of elimination of excess *pitta* from the body is via the urinary tract. Here cooling diuretics like coriander, dandelion, *punarnava*, or *gokshura* can be used. There are many safe and effective diuretic herbs that contain tonic properties and are rich in potassium and other minerals, but caution should be used when taking diuretics over extended periods, because they can be drying to the body and cause electrolyte imbalances. (See Diuretics.)

Excess *pitta* can also be eliminated through the skin as in the case of superficial fever due to a cold, flu, or mild infection. In this case, diaphoretics (herbs that promote sweating) can help bring the temperature down. If there is high fever, cooling diaphoretic herbs like boneset, coriander, *guduchi*, or yarrow work well, while warm diaphoretics such as *tulsi* or ginger can increase *pitta*. Antipyretic herbs, which are extremely cold and bitter, act deeply to decrease the temperature too, especially in deep seated or intermittent fever. As a general rule, if a fever is higher than 103 degrees, antipyretic herbs should be used. Many alterative herbs, such as *kutki* (gentian), goldenseal, or barberry have also an antipyretic action.

Rashes, hives, psoriasis, and other inflammatory skin eruptions are related to the hot, liquid, and spreading qualities of *pitta* in the *rasa* (plasma) and *rakta* (blood) *dhatus*. Here alterative herbs, which are typically cold and bitter, are often the medicine of choice, but one should not forget to keep a holistic approach. There is a huge emotional and immunological component to chronic skin diseases like eczema and psoriasis that needs to be explored. Just blindly treating these types of conditions with cold, bitter herbs may not be effective and over time can weaken the digestion and dry or deplete the bodily tissues. Cooling nervines like *brahmi* and skullcap, both of which also have alterative properties, are perfect for cooling and calming the volatile *pitta* emotions, as well as clearing heat from the blood and liver. High *pitta* in the *rasa* and *rakta dhatus* may also cause bleeding disorders, sores, and ulcers. In those cases, astringent herbs, which are usually cooling, are also helpful to stop bleeding, bind, and promote healing of those tissues.

Kapha Management (*Kapha Pakrama*)

Kapha, deriving mainly from the water and earth elements, has heavy, cool, static, wet, dense, soft, and cloudy qualities. *Kapha* is anabolic by nature and is managed with reducing and scraping (*lechana*) herbs and therapies. Warming and drying herbs and foods are most beneficial to counter its cold and damp qualities. The main tastes for pacifying *kapha* are pungent, bitter, and astringent. Being more sedentary by nature, *kapha* responds well to increased activity and a varied routine.

The main tissue associated with *kapha* is *rasa dhatu*, which contains more than 90% water. Because of its water element, diuretic therapy is a good way to promote the removal of *kleda*, the liquid component of *kapha* in the body, through the urinary system. Another way to dispel excess *kapha* is to purify *rasa dhatu* by promoting sweating with warming diaphoretic herbs like ginger, *ajwan*, or *tulsi*.

One of the main therapies used in Ayurveda for removing excess *kapha* is *vamana*, or emetic therapy. *Vamana* is very effective at removing *kapha* that has accumulated in the upper regions of the body, specifically the stomach and respiratory tract. This therapy is usually part of *Panchakarma*, which is a more involved cleansing program where excess *kapha* is coaxed out from the deeper tissues and then moved into the stomach. If *kapha* is in the lower parts of the torso, vomiting is contraindicated. In this case, purgation (*virechana*) or enema (*basti*) therapies are used.

Kapha types tend to have a slow and sluggish digestive fire (*manda agni*), so hot pungent herbs can help to kindle *agni* and burn fat and *ama* in the body. Many of these pungent herbs are also used as culinary spices, such as ginger, *ajwan*, black pepper, or cayenne. Pungent herbs also have carminative properties that help to dispel gas, which can form as a result of sluggish digestion, or when *kapha* or *ama* obstruct the normal movement of *vata*.

Phlegm is associated with *kapha* and is also the waste product formed by the *rasa dhatu*. One of the signs of excess *kapha* is heaviness in the stomach, which is caused by excess phlegm in the stomach. *Kapha* can spread from its main sites (stomach and lungs) and lodge anywhere in the body, causing abnormal growths like lipomas, fibroids, cysts, and generally benign fatty tumors.

Causative Factors of Toxic Formation

In Ayurveda, one of the primary causes of disease is the formation of *ama*, which is the accumulation of toxins, or improperly digested food. When the digestive fire is low, due to *doshic* derangement, improper food combining, overeating, and so on, the food precursors remain in the GI tract. These poorly digested food precursors, or *ama*, get absorbed into the general circulation and eventually deposit themselves into the tissues, organs, and channels of the body, leading to imbalance and disease.

Some schools of thought believe that a disturbed *dosha* can become *ama* as well. Furthermore, when the bodily wastes (i.e. urine, feces, and sweat) are not eliminated properly, they cause *ama* to accumulate in the body. Too much *ama* can give way to lethargy, low appetite, lack of strength, mental confusion, restlessness, and a feeling of heaviness and general fatigue.

If *agni* is low at the level of a tissue element, it can cause *ama* to form in that particular *dhatu* as a result of poorly developed tissue. For example, if there is low *agni* at the level of *meda dhatu*, the fat tissue, then too much fat can form there.

Ama and *agni* have opposite qualities. *Ama* is heavy, sticky, dense, cloudy, gross, slimy, damp, cold, impure, and foul smelling, and tends to suppress the power of *agni*. *Agni*, on the other hand, is light, hot, dry, clear, subtle, pure, and fragrant. If *agni* becomes impaired, *ama* can form; conversely, if *ama* is allowed to accumulate, *agni* will eventually become diminished.

Excessive intake of sweet, sour, and salty foods, all of which are heavy and cause dampness, can eventually weaken *agni*, thus promoting *ama* formation. Sweet taste, which is composed of earth and water, is heavy, cold, and sweet. Salty taste, primarily made up of fire and water, is heavy and wet. Sour taste is created with earth and fire. Salty and sour tastes increase both *ama* and heat in the body, which is commonly seen in conditions such as fevers, inflammation, and boggy infections.

Doshas and *Ama*

An important factor for understanding the nature of any condition is detecting whether or not *ama* is present along with the vitiated *dosha*. When *ama* is associated with a *dosha,* it is referred to as *sama* (*sa* means "with"). If there is no *ama* associated with the *dosha,* it is referred to as *nirama* (*nir* means "without").

When a *dosha* becomes provoked it can easily disturb the normal functions of *agni*, causing *ama* to form along with it. This often starts in the main site of that particular *dosha*, that is, *vata* in the colon, *pitta* in the small intestine, and *kapha* in the lungs and stomach, but *ama dosha* can also move into and affect any of the bodily tissues.

Whenever *ama* is present along with the *dosha*, the focus is to first reduce *ama* and prevent its formation. So, depending on the situation, various herbs can be chosen according to their properties, energies, and tastes. Herbs of choice should be those that do *deepana*, or kindling of the digestive fire, and *pachana*, or burning of *ama*.

Bitter herbs such as alteratives and bitter tonics, which are composed of air and ether, can help to neutralize and break down toxins. These are best used for *pitta* and *kapha* conditions, and can often be combined with warm pungent herbs to balance out their cold quality. Pungent tasting herbs like ginger or black pepper, composed of fire and air, are the best to kindle *agni* and burn *ama*. Carminative herbs like cumin and fennel help to redirect or regulate the movement of *vata* within the GI tract, thus improving the digestion and absorption, as well as the elimination of *ama*. As a result, they help to relieve gas, bloating, and abdominal pain associated with the presence of toxins, which can also be removed with laxative and purgative substances.

Often pacifying *dosha* and reducing toxins can be done simultaneously, but if there is much *ama* present, the emphasis should first be placed on clearing it. When *dosha* is mixed with *ama* it can take on a different manifestation than the usual appearance of the *dosha*. For example, *vata*, which is usually cold, dry, and light, can appear to be heavy and damp when *ama* is associated with it. Likewise, *pitta* is usually hot, sharp, light, and oily, but it can become cold, heavy, and damp due to the presence of *ama*. Furthermore, *kapha*, which shares similar qualities with *ama*, is already heavy and slow. Therefore, when it is mixed with *ama* it becomes even more prone to accumulation and stagnation.

In general, when a *dosha* is increased, herbs that possess opposite qualities to that *dosha* are used to facilitate balance. For example, excess cold in the body is treated with heating herbs and therapies. But in a *sama* condition, where the *dosha* is mixed with *ama*, the choice of herbs needs to address both aspects and balance them out. Herbs that often pacify the *dosha* may aggravate the condition, due to the presence of *ama*, and herbs that generally provoke the *dosha* may be indicated. For instance, cooling herbs, which usually pacify *pitta*, may contribute to the accumulation of *ama* because they can eventually weaken *agni*, whereas heating herbs that usually provoke *pitta* can provide relief due to their ability to kindle *agni* and burn *ama*. For this reason, we must not only determine the *dosha* involved, but also whether it is *sama* or *nirama*, with or without toxins, and balance the treatment accordingly.

As already mentioned, pungent tasting herbs help to burn *ama* while bitter herbs help to neutralize it, break it up, and aid in its elimination. Astringent herbs can have a mixed effect. When taken in moderation and combined with pungent and bitter herbs, they can help to mend tissues damaged by *ama*, but in excess they can cause constriction of the membranes, making the body tighten its grip on *ama*.

The first line of approach should be to remove *ama* without further aggravating the *doshas* involved. For example, in a *sama pitta* condition, heating digestive stimulant and carminative herbs can be used in larger amounts and gradually reduced. Once the clearing of *ama* is accomplished, a more constitutional treatment, focused on balancing the *doshas*, can be undertaken.

Indications of *Sama* and *Nirama*

The indications below are intended to give an idea of the various symptoms that may arise in the case of *sama dosha* or *nirama dosha* conditions.

Vata

Indications of *sama vata*: Coated tongue, foul smelling flatulence, breath, and feces; constipation, abdominal cramping and distention, vague pain (especially in the abdominal area), low appetite, feeling of heaviness, weakness, aggravated by oil massage; palpation, slow pulse; pain in the tendons, ligaments, and joints; frozen joints. Symptoms get aggravated in cloudy and rainy weather.

Sama *vata* has an affinity to the musculoskeletal system. Long standing *ama* can also cause rheumatoid arthritis, osteoarthritis, sciatica, and lumbago.

Treatment includes: Carminative and stimulant herbs like cumin and fennel, warming pungent herbs such as fresh ginger to burn *ama*, laxatives, and purgatives like *haritaki* to eliminate toxins. Specific Ayurvedic compounds such as *hingwastak churna, ama pachak bati, simhanad guggulu,* or *yogaraj guggulu* are also helpful for a variety of *sama vata* related disorders.

Indications of *nirama vata*: No distention, constipation, or foul odors; clear tongue; mild pain, relieved by massage; less fatigue; dry mouth with astringent taste; dry skin, decreased body weight, and emaciation.

Note: *Nirama vata* conditions can be more destructive because *vata* is subtle and dry, and can penetrate more directly, deeply, and quickly into the tissues. *Nirama vata* can also move into the bone tissue causing degenerative arthritis.

Treatment includes: Mainly anabolic herbs that possess sweet, heavy, and moistening qualities like nutritive and rejuvenating tonics to counter degeneration. *Mahayogaraj guggulu* is effective in degenerative types of arthritis.

Pitta

Indications of *sama pitta*: Loss of appetite, little thirst, heaviness in the stomach, nausea, bilious vomiting, bad breath, bitter or sour taste in the mouth, heartburn, hyperacidity; rashes, ulcers; bruises easily, bleeding disorders; yellow coating on the tongue, yellow urine, yellow or green feces and mucus; cloudy perception. Symptoms may be aggravated by cold.

Note: The digestive secretions in the stomach are a component of *pitta dosha*. If there are excess gastric secretions, the excess liquid quality of *pitta* can weaken the gastric fire, thus promoting the formation of *ama*.

Treatment includes: Mainly bitter and pungent herbs to clear toxins. Herbs that have both a sweet and bitter taste like *shatavari* can also be used, and stronger bitters like *neem*, barberry, or bitter compounds like *mahasudarshan* are extremely effective to dispel *ama*. Even though hot, pungent tasting herbs are typically *pitta* aggravating, here they may be necessary initially to rekindle *agni*. They can be balanced with cooling bitter herbs to make a good *pitta* digestive tonic. A good example of a compound that has both a warming and cooling herbs that is used for *sama pitta* conditions is *avipattikara churna*.

Indications of *nirama pitta*: Strong appetite and thirst but poor digestion and absorption (due to high *pitta* burning foodstuff); dizziness, giddiness; irritability, burning sensations, hot flashes, red or inflamed tongue with less coating than *sama pitta*.

Note: Without *ama, pitta* can easily penetrate into the body and destroy the tissues. It can eventually create irritation, perforated ulcers, and even hemorrhage.

Treatment includes: Mainly sweet, cooling, and bitter herbs. Tonic herbs like *shatavari, vidari, guduchi,* and licorice are helpful. The Ayurvedic compounds *kama dudha* and *gulwel sattwa* (the starchy extract of *guduchi*) are also very useful.

Kapha

Indications of *sama kapha*: Dull, aching and generalized pain; fatigue, general heaviness; thick, white coating on the tongue; low appetite, heaviness in the stomach; thick and sticky mucus, thread-like saliva, mucus in stools; tightness in the chest, difficult breathing.

Treatment includes: Stimulating, pungent, and bitter herbs mainly to decongest phlegm and burn and clear toxins. The main compound used for *sama kapha* conditions is *trikatu churna*.

Note: *Kapha* is already heavy, slow moving and fairly static in nature, so the presence of *ama*, which is also heavy, slows *kapha* to a stand still.

Indications of *nirama kapha*: Watery or frothy mucus, mucus drains easily, normal appetite, clear tongue, no mucus in stool, clear urine, no pain, sweet taste in mouth.

Treatment includes: Pungent and sweet herbs that help to remove excess phlegm, *ama*, and *kapha*.

Health and Disease

Ayurveda defines health as the state where all aspects of a person are working properly and harmoniously together. That is, the digestive fire (*agni*) is in a balanced condition; the three *doshas* are in equilibrium according to the individual constitution; waste products (*malas*) are produced and eliminated normally; and the mind, senses, and consciousness are working in harmony. When the balance of any of these aspects becomes disturbed, disease can manifest. In other words, imbalance and illness are the result of living out of harmony with the original individual constitution.

Disease is the end result of a long process that can be prevented, detected, and addressed at any stage. This process begins when the *doshas* become disturbed. Temporary disturbances are common and normal, but further problems may arise if these are left to linger and are not corrected. As previously stated, each healthy *dosha* is at home in a main area—*vata* in the colon, *pitta* in the small intestine, and *kapha* in the stomach. These are the primary sites from which each *dosha* manifests and spreads its influence.

***Vata, pitta,* and *kapha* are constantly going through cycles of change in three stages:** Accumulation, aggravation, and pacification. For example, *pitta* begins to accumulate in the late spring, gets aggravated in the hot summer, and then becomes naturally pacified when the weather cools in the fall. If the increased *dosha* isn't pacified naturally through a change in season, it undergoes further changes and disease may result. So, if *kapha* increases during the cold winter months, but returns to normal soon after, disease will not develop. If, say, *kapha* is further aggravated, it will move into the general circulation and spread into the deep tissues, where it will generate pathological changes. Then disease will develop. In this case, an aggravated *dosha* leaves its site, enters the general circulation, and lodges in a tissue, disturbing the nature, structure, and function of that *dhatu*. This whole process is the pathogenesis of disease.

Typically, *vata* diseases begin in the colon, *pitta* ailments in the small intestine, and *kapha* problems in the upper part of the stomach, although there are exceptions to this. Obviously, we can all aid the process of restoring balance by following the appropriate diet and lifestyle in accordance with each season and/or *dosha* imbalance.

In Ayurveda, the pathogenesis of disease is called *samprapti*, which literally means "the birth of pain." There are six stages of *samprapti*: Accumulation (*sanchaya*), provocation (*prakopa*), spread (*prasara*), deposition or localization (*sthana samsraya*), manifestation (*vyakti*), and destruction of tissues and complications (*bheda*). Exploring these stages is beyond the scope of this book, but becoming aware of this process can help to understand that any disease is the end result of a process that can be detected, counteracted, and treated at different stages. Furthermore, if we listen to the early warnings that the inner intelligence of the body sends in the form of signs and symptoms, and act upon them appropriately and according to Ayurvedic principles, then we can increase the chances of avoiding further imbalance and complications.

Ayurveda states that the key to a healthy life ultimately lies within each person, and encourages us all to become more in touch with our inner voice of intuition instead of blindly following the cravings and unhealthy habits created by the mind. Emotions can affect our body just as much as what we eat affects our emotions. If we feel happy, every cell in our body becomes happy and revitalized. Likewise, if we are sad, angry, or frustrated, these feeling are reflected in the entire organism and weaken it over time.

Ultimately, disease has its roots in the false notion that the infinite, pure consciousness is limited to the confines of the body and mind. This is not to say that one who has attained inner peace will never experience physical disease, or that physical health cannot be experienced by one who hasn't. Both health and disease are aspects of life. The difference lies in *how* they are experienced.

It is difficult to be healthy if stress, anger, and anxiety are constantly sapping the vital energy. This is why Ayurveda places great emphasis not only on the physical aspects of health, but also on daily routines (*dinacharya*) and spiritual practices such as yoga, meditation, prayer (or worship), mindfulness, and self-inquiry. Furthermore, these kinds of practices possess a medicinal power that rejuvenates the whole being. Learning to live a more peaceful, yogic type of life can most certainly help us to maintain optimal health and prevent disease.

In Ayurveda, as in the yogic traditions, ultimate health is the state in which the individual self abides in its true nature. In other words, when the individual *prana* merges with the Cosmic *Prana*. In this state, the light of pure consciousness shines fully within the *buddhi*, or intelligence sheath. This is possible when the mind is stabilized through the practice of meditation.

The Importance of Diet & Lifestyle

There is no better support to any herbal regime than adhering to a healthy diet and lifestyle, especially when it is specific to the constitution and present imbalances. Just relying on herbs to restore harmony of body, mind, and consciousness is not enough in the long run. If the habits that cause imbalance are not understood and uprooted, they will always present obstacles in the path of healing. An analogy that comes to mind would be washing your clothes in muddy water and expect them to come clean.

As stated in the ancient texts, it is much easier to maintain health than it is to cure disease. Most people tend to not pay attention to their habits and addictions, nor do they heed the signs and symptoms of imbalance until these have become a "disease." Then they want a quick fix to suppress those symptoms without ever getting to the root cause of their disorders. This cycle can only go on for so long before they are forced to deal with more serious conditions.

This is why when studying the benefits that herbs play in the process of *doshic* management it is important to also remember how important food is in this process. After all, food is medicine too, and one we get more of than any other, so it has an enormous impact on our overall health. Even if the herbal treatment is right, it may still miss its mark if the diet and lifestyle are not supportive to the healing process.

From an Ayurvedic perspective, one of the main keys to optimal health is to help the body eliminate toxins and to reestablish constitutional balance. To achieve this, Ayurveda emphasizes the importance of proper nutrition, food combining, and cooking methods, as well as herbal nutrition, all based on the specific needs of the individual and any current imbalance of the *doshas*.

For optimum nutrition, it is best to choose food that is organic, fresh, and locally grown, whenever possible. In Ayurveda food, drinks, and spices are categorized according to their taste (sweet, salty, sour, bitter, pungent, and astringent), the energetic effect they have on the *doshas*, as well as their post-digestive effect on the tissues. This is why when choosing foods it is important to understand the original constitution so as to choose foods that have the opposite qualities to those that are already predominant in the constitution. Furthermore, understanding the current state of the *doshas* is also crucial for making the right food choices.

Many of the spices used in Ayurvedic cooking, such as turmeric, ginger, cumin, fenugreek, coriander, and cardamom, amongst others, are also medicinal herbs used in Ayurvedic herbology. Cooking daily with those spices can greatly enhance digestion, absorption, and assimilation of food, improve the appetite and elimination, nourish the internal organs, and prevent *doshic* imbalance. Spices also provide a harmonious blend of the six tastes. Taste is medicinal and is the first form of nourishment. A meal containing a balanced blend of all six tastes, aside from being more appealing to the tongue, is also more digestible at a deep cellular level.

Modern research is now validating the benefits of many of the herbs and spices used in Ayurvedic cooking. Turmeric, for instance, is highly effective in the treatment of type 2 diabetes, skin diseases, infections, and hepatic and inflammatory disorders. Cumin, coriander, fennel, nutmeg, and cardamom are extremely helpful in the treatment of a wide variety of digestive complaints, as is ginger for the treatment of respiratory congestion, fevers, and colds. There are literally thousands of medicinal uses to such spices.

Another vital aspect of Ayurvedic nutrition is proper food combining. In Ayurveda not all foods are compatible. When eaten or cooked together, certain foods can disturb the normal function of the digestive fire and promote the accumulation of toxins in the body. Various factors, such as the taste, qualities, and energies of foods, as well as how long they take to digest, affect how they combine. Heavy foods such as whole grains, dairy, meats, and starches don't combine well with light foods like fruit, which digest quicker. Ayurveda places great emphasis on the art of food combining and encourages us all to take responsibility for our health as much as possible by making appropriate diet and lifestyle changes. What we eat and how we live on a daily basis can be our strongest allies in restoring and maintaining health. All other therapeutic measures will be strongly supported by this daily effort.

Along with a balanced diet, incorporating other healthy habits into a daily routine can prevent imbalance at its very root. A lifestyle that integrates regular eating and sleeping habits will bring discipline and help maintain the harmony of the *doshas*, thus promoting overall good health. An Ayurvedic clinician can provide dietary and lifestyle guidelines as well as herbal nutrition that is more specific to the individual constitution, *doshic* imbalance, and situation of each person. However, Ayurveda offers some basic dietary guidelines that can benefit everyone's health. For instance, it is important to eat at appropriate times of the day in accordance with the natural rhythm of the body. The most substantial meal is best eaten between 11 a.m. and noon. Since this is often difficult, one should at least try to eat bigger meals in the daytime and smaller meals at night, preferably before 7 p.m., so that the food can be digested before going to sleep.

Ayurveda discourages eating on the go and at odd hours of the day. The following guideline should be matched as best as possible: Breakfast before 8 a.m.; lunch between 11 a.m. and 1 p.m.; and dinner between 5 and 7 p.m. It is important to allow 5-6 hours between meals for complete digestion. People with a strong digestion and raging appetite can have a light snack, such as fruit, juice, or nuts between meals to maintain energy. To assure that we get the most from the food we ingest it is important not to overeat. It takes our brain about 15 to 20 minutes to acknowledge that the stomach is full, so self-control is the key here. We must discipline ourselves to stop eating before feeling sated. A stomach gorged with food weakens the entire digestive process and causes indigestion and accumulation of *ama* in the GI tract.

Because foods have different qualities and require different digestive energies, food combining is of the utmost importance in Ayurveda. For instance, fruits digest quicker than grains, so eating the two together confuses the digestive process and creates fermentation and *ama*. When a food that digests easily and quickly (such as fruit) is made to stick around in the stomach while other, heavier foods (such as grains and carbohydrates) finish their "cooking process," a mixed message that disrupts the *agni* is sent to the internal organs. Foods that have a predominantly sour quality, or fermented foods such as yogurt, should not be eaten with sweet foods like milk or fruit. The sour quality can cause the milk to separate and ferment in the stomach, leading to toxic buildup in the GI tract and the deeper tissues over time.

Drinking too much water while eating can wash away digestive enzymes and weaken the digestive fire. However, sipping on a cup of water at room temperature while eating benefits the break down of food and aids the digestive process. The following guidelines are not exhaustive and are mentioned here for educational purposes.

A trained Ayurvedic clinician can recommend an appropriate diet based on nutritional values, constitution, seasons, age, and individual health conditions.

Incompatible Food Combining

Do Not Eat	With
Milk	Bananas, fish, meat, melons, sour fruits, *kitchari* (rice and mung bean porridge), yeasted breads, cherries, yogurt
Melons	Grains, starches, fried foods, dairy products
Starches	Eggs, dairy, bananas, dates, most fruits
Honey	An equal amount (by weight) of *ghee*, or when it's been boiled or cooked
Radishes	Milk, bananas, raisins
Nightshades (potato, tomato, eggplant)	Yogurt, milk, melons, cucumber
Yogurt	Milk, sour fruits, melons
Hot drinks	Meat, fish, mangoes, starches, cheese
Eggs	Milk, meat, fish, yogurt, melons, cheese, fish, bananas
Fruit	Any other food
Corn	Dates, raisins, bananas
Lemon	Yogurt, milk, cucumbers, tomatoes

General Eating Habits to Avoid:

Overeating;

Eating food that you can't digest;

Eating soon after a full meal;

Eating when constipated;

Eating without hunger;

Eating incompatible food combinations;

Eating at the wrong time of day;

Eating too much heavy food or too little light food;

Drinking cold or chilled water;

Drinking fruit juice or eating fruit with meals;

Too much water or no water during a meal;

Snacking between meals;

Emotional eating.

Along with a balanced diet, incorporating other healthy habits into a daily routine can prevent disease at its very root. Ayurveda refers to this daily routine as *dinacharya*, which is the art of living in awareness with every activity of the day. In this context, a seemingly mundane act can become a mindful meditation. A lifestyle that incorporates regular eating and sleeping habits, as well as a balanced daily routine, will bring discipline and help maintain the harmony of the *doshas,* thus promoting overall good health. The following are general *dinacharya* guidelines.

Waste products should be eliminated from the body first thing in the morning. This helps to revitalize the organism and prepare the body to receive more nutrients. According to Ayurveda, you should have at least one complete bowel movement a day. If not, the toxins can be reabsorbed into the tissues. To prevent this, it is important to eat enough fiber-rich food and good quality oils, such as *ghee*, flax, olive, or sesame oil, and avoid excessive amounts of raw foods and chilled drinks. There are traditional herbal compounds that help restore and maintain the tone of the colon while gently cleansing it on a daily basis. Be careful not to abuse laxatives, since even the herbal ones can weaken the tone of the colon and create dependency.

Another early morning Ayurvedic practice is to gently brush the teeth and scrape the tongue. A thick coating on the tongue indicates that there is *ama* from improperly digested food in the GI tract. You should scrape off this coating with a metallic tongue scraper seven times prior to brushing your teeth.

Early morning bathing is another basic *dinacharya* practice. In yogic traditions, bathing symbolizes the purification of the soul. It also washes the sweat residue from the pores of the skin, leaving a healthy radiant glow. Gentle herbal soaps or powders can be use to cleanse the skin. The daily practice of rubbing the body with oil can further nourish the skin and deeper tissues. This can be performed before or after showering. *Vata* constitutions should use sesame oil; *pitta* should use coconut oil; and *kapha* are best with corn oil.

As much as possible, you should wake before sunrise for meditation. In the Vedic tradition, the pre dawn hours are known as *Brahma murta*. This quiet, calm time, when the Earth and its inhabitants are still asleep, is most conducive to a meditation practice. Even if it cannot be done before dawn, regular meditation is essential for the maintenance of health. Actually, there is no better medicine than meditation. It helps to clear the mind, making it more placid and peaceful, and helps to rejuvenate and purify the entire nervous system. If we are more peaceful, then our own healing energy and awareness increase. It may also be beneficial to add an herb or two to help rejuvenate the mind. After all, the content of our consciousness is constantly being reflected within the physical body.

Yoga and exercise are also important healthy habits. The type of exercise you choose should be suitable for your specific constitution and not in excess. Brisk walking is probably the best exercise for all constitutions, as is traditional hatha yoga. This will stimulate the digestive fire, balance organ functions, reduce stress, and relieve constipation. *Kapha* individuals can perform the most vigorous type of exercise. *Pitta* people should do exercise with medium intensity and ideally during the coolest times of the day. Those with a *vata* constitution should do exercise slowly with an emphasis on mindfulness. Even though *vata* types often love to jog, better choices are yoga, walking, swimming, stretching, and t'ai chi. Some strength training with weights can also be helpful to keep the muscles toned. Relaxation and sound sleep will result in good health, as the body rejuvenates when it is relaxed.

Finally, cultivating clear, compassionate, and loving relationships is another important aspect of a healthy lifestyle. Suppressed or unresolved emotions can poison the body just as much as bad food combining. Regular meditation can enhance awareness of relationships and promote discrimination as well.

PART III: HERBAL MEDICINE

Actions and Classification of Herbs

Alterative Herbs (*Rakta Shodhana Karma*)

In Ayurveda, alterative herbs are categorized as having *rakta shodhana,* or blood cleansing properties. These herbs have a direct effect upon the liver and spleen, which are considered the roots of the blood and plasma channels (*raktavaha srotas* and *rasavaha srotas*), but many have accompanying properties that act upon the lungs, kidneys, skin, and digestive tract. They promote a natural healing response resulting from the cleansing of the body's overall terrain. They aid in purifying the lymphatic tissue and increasing the white blood cell count. They are effectively used for treating skin eruptions, high fevers, herpes, boils, venereal and other infections, cancer, arthritis, and gout.

Typically, alteratives are bitter and have a cooling action, although some are heating. They are valuable for their anti-inflammatory, antibacterial, and antibiotic effects. They are gentler on the body than standard antibiotic drugs, but they too can aggravate *vata* and weaken the digestive fire when used in excess.

Cooling alteratives can be combined with heating alteratives to help balance and strengthen their detoxifying action. Pungent alteratives are hot, helping to stimulate the digestive fire, burn *ama*, resolve fever, increase circulation, and break up blood clots. They are also valuable in ridding the body of parasites and worms.

> **Some cooling alteratives are:** Aloe vera, blue flag, burdock, chaparral, dandelion, echinacea, gentian, *guduchi, manjista, neem*, plantain, poke root, red clover, red sandalwood, sarsaparilla, white sandalwood, wild indigo, and yellow dock.
>
> **Some hot, pungent alteratives are:** *Ajwan*, asafoetida, bayberry, black pepper, cayenne, cinnamon, clove, garlic, ginger, prickly ash, and wild ginger.

Anthelmintic or Antiparasitical Herbs (*Krumighna Karma*)

Anthelmintics are substances that help to eliminate worms and other parasites. In Ayurveda, this category of herbs is referred to as *krumighna karma.* The Sanskrit term *krumi* refers to worms, but all other parasites (fungal and bacterial) or yeast infections, as well as some viral infections carried by insects have a similar effect on the the body as *krumi*.

Ayurveda views parasitic conditions from a *doshic* perspective. When a *dosha* gets aggravated it can disturb the digestive fire, giving way to the formation of *ama* due to improperly digested food. This *ama* takes on the qualities of the excess *dosha* creating a welcoming environment to parasites that share a similar nature. This is why proper diet and lifestyle, along with good hygiene, are very important when dealing with *krumi* conditions.

Parasites arising from excess *kapha* have an affinity to mucus and phlegm and tend to originate in the stomach and move through the intestines, or can also reside in the lungs. They can cause nausea, indigestion, loss of appetite, excess salivation, giddiness, flatulence, emaciation, sinus congestion, and nasal crust and irritation.

Pitta types of *krumi* have an affinity to and lodge in the blood and sweat. Symptoms include burning and itching sensations, hair loss, fungal infections, skin discoloration, raised patches of skin, and a variety of skin ailments, including leprosy, as well as some diseases carried by mosquitoes, fleas, and ticks.

Vata types of parasites take up residence in the intestines. They usually move downward, but when they increase in number they can also move upward to the small intestine and stomach, causing stomach pain and the breath to smell like feces. These *krumi* can also cause dryness of the skin and feces, constipation, weakness, loss of appetite, and itching of the anus.

Cooling and bitter anthelmintic herbs like black walnut, goldenseal, grapefruit seed extract, *kutaja*, *neem*, papaya seeds, pomegranate, *shardunika*, and wormwood neutralize *ama* and pacify *pitta*, so they work well for treating *pitta* types of *krumi*.

Heating anthelmintics such as *ajwan*, asafoetida, cayenne, clove, garlic, pennyroyal, prickly ash, pumpkin seeds, rue, *vidanga*, and wormseed kindle *agni* and burn *ama* and parasites, so they are useful for *vata* types of *krumi*.

Since *kapha* is reduced by bitter, pungent, and astringent tastes, *kapha* types of *krumi* can be treated with herbs from both categories.

In acute situations, or when there is not a clear understanding of which *doshas* are involved, combining several anthelmintic herbs can help to create a broad-spectrum formula for a quick and powerful action. In chronic or dormant parasitical conditions, adding a small amount of one or two herbs to a more constitutionally supportive formula is easier on the system and helps to send a subtle but constant message to the parasites to move out.

Some anthelmintics like *neem* tend to deplete the bodily tissues, especially the sperm; hence they should not be used in large doses or by themselves for extended periods of time. Careful consideration should be taken in choosing the appropriate anthelmintic herbs and dosage, depending on the severity of the case, the individual constitution, and underline cause and *doshic* imbalance, as well as the nature of the parasites and length of treatment.

Anti-Microbial Herbs

Anti-microbial herbs help to strengthen the body's natural defense mechanisms against pathogenic microorganisms. To some degree, this action may be due to certain active constituents present in a particular herb. For example, in the case of echinacea, the constituent echinacien is viewed as being responsible for the herb's antibacterial action. There is some truth to this without a doubt, but whole herbs contain many constituents as well as other qualities, tastes, and energies that contribute to its usefulness. It is important to remember that herbs always act as a synergistic whole.

Herbs that have anti-microbial properties are also categorized as anti-fungal, antiseptic, anthelmintic (anti-parasitical), and antiviral, and are often *pitta* reducing. Many anti-inflammatory, alterative, and antipyretic herbs have some anti-microbial properties too, including heating and pungent herbs like cayenne, turmeric, and garlic.

This group of herbs is sometimes referred to as being antibiotic, but this is not entirely accurate from a holistic point of view. Anti-microbial herbs help augment the natural healing power of the body against infections and such, but they do so in a gentler manner than antibiotic drugs, which tend to stress the internal organs and disturb the digestive fire and intestinal flora, often leaving one more predisposed to reoccurring infection. Certain cold, bitter herbs like goldenseal, for instance, can also weaken the digestion and disturb the intestinal flora if they are used in excess or for long periods of time, but to a far lesser degree.

When choosing from this category, it is important to select herbs that have an affinity to the particular organ or system that is being treated. For example, clove and osha root can be used for respiratory complaints, since they also have an affinity to the lungs. Bitter herbs like gentian and *guduchi* will act directly on the blood as well as the digestive tract. Likewise, herbs like calendula, *manjista,* and *neem* are helpful for skin ailments.

Antipyretic Herbs and Bitter Tonics

In Western herbalism bitter tonics, also called bitters, are thought to stimulate and improve the appetite and digestion, and to increase the elimination of toxins and waste products from the body, thereby helping to purify the blood. They are considered to help invigorate, strengthen, and tonify the organs and have been used for treating convalescence from disease and run-down conditions.

From an Ayurvedic perspective, strong bitters are not considered tonics because they are extremely cold, drying, and reducing to the bodily tissues. Therefore, they are used with caution or not at all in deficient conditions. When used in excess, they can aggravate *vata*, thus causing dryness of the colon and constipation, as well as weaken the tissues, the digestive fire, and tone of the GI tract. Ayurveda is not opposed to the idea that bitter herbs can help to stimulate the digestive fire, but considers that their action is quick and temporary, and that over time they can actually weaken the digestion.

This category of herbs would be more appropriate for the treatment of *pitta* related digestive disorders to reduce acidity and bile production, as well as to promote the elimination of toxins and excess heat from the body. Much the same as alterative herbs, they help to pacify *pitta* and regulate normal functions of the liver and spleen, and often play a key role in the treatment of hepatic disorders. In a sense, they could be viewed as being *pitta* tonics.

Bitter herbs also have antipyretic properties and are especially useful for *pitta jwara*, or *pitta* related fevers that have moved into the liver, blood, or other deep tissues of the body. In such conditions there may be symptoms of nausea, high temperature (over 103 degrees), fainting, unquenchable thirst, bitter and sour tasting vomit, sweating, inflammation, and infection. They do not suppress the fever, but work by clearing heat and eliminating the toxins that cause the fever. For this reason, they can also be used to treat hepatitis, pneumonia, and intermittent or malarial type of fevers.

In acute conditions of fever, such as the first onset of colds or the flu, it is better to use diaphoretic herbs that promote the dilation of surface capillaries, open the skin pores, induce sweating, and restore circulation, thus helping to dispel chills and other pernicious influences causing the fever.

Bitter taste is composed of the air and ether elements. It has light and dry qualities and a catabolic activity, hence it helps to burn excess fat and *ama* from the body, and is very effective in treating a variety of *kapha* disorders, including obesity and adult onset diabetes.

Bitters like barberry, *neem*, and turmeric are useful to regulate pancreatic function and sugar metabolism, as they have proven to be quite effective for controlling blood sugar levels.

> **Examples of antipyretic herbs and bitters:** Aloe vera, barberry, chaparral, *chitrak*, dandelion leaf, gentian, goldenseal, *guduchi*, *kutki*, *neem*, Oregon grape root, and white poplar.

According to Ayurveda, bitter herbs like barberry, *guduchi*, or Oregon grape are considered to possess a warm energy, and they can be combined with warming pungent herbs like cardamom, ginger, and *pippali* to kindle the digestive fire without aggravating *pitta*. This approach is good for *sama pitta* conditions.

Aphrodisiac Herbs (*Vajikarana*)

Aphrodisiac herbs help to nourish and stimulate the sexual organs and tissues. In Sanskrit, *vaji* means "horse" and *karana* means "power," so *vajikarana* conveys the idea of the power or strength of a horse. In Ayurvedic pharmacology, some are categorized as *shukrala*, or herbs that aid in increasing spermatogenesis in the male. Those that have an affinity to the female reproductive tissue are known as *artala*. These improve the health of the ovum, promote menstruation and lactation, and maintain the growth and tone of the mastic tissue.

The term aphrodisiac often conveys the idea of a substance that simply increases the libido. Although this is true, some aphrodisiac herbs also possess similar properties to *rasayana* herbs or nutritive tonics, in that they help to rejuvenate all bodily tissues. Furthermore, because they nourish the reproductive tissues, they also help to increase *ojas*, which is the essence of all bodily tissues that can be transformed into spiritual energy. In yoga, *ojas* is vital to support concentration and enhance spiritual practices such as meditation.

Vajikarana herbs can be categorized as stimulants and tonics. Stimulants are typically heating and *rajasic* (energizing, active), like damiana, fenugreek, and garlic, so they help to decrease *kapha* and have more of an invigorating action on the sexual organs. Tonics, whether warming or cooling, are more nourishing and help to restore the overall quality and quantity of tissues. Keep in mind that many herbs have both a tonic and stimulating action in greater or lesser degrees.

Some aphrodisiac herbs are warming, such as *ashwagandha*, and are best for pacifying *vata*, while others are cooling, like *shatavari* and wild yam, and help to pacify *pitta*. Because many of these herbs are heavy and sweet they tend to diminish *agni* and increase *kapha* and *ama*, but they may be used along with warming and spicy herbs to help in their digestion.

Examples of stimulating *vajikaranas*: Asafoetida, clove, damiana, fenugreek, garlic, *pippali*, raw onion, and *shilajit*.

Examples of *vajikarana* tonics: Angelica (tang kuei), *ashwagandha*, *bala*, fo-ti, *ghee*, ginseng, *gokshura*, kapi kacchu (*atmagupta*), licorice, lotus seeds, marshmallow, onion, saw palmetto, sesame seeds, *shatavari*, Solomon's seal, sugar, saffron, *vidari*, and wild yam.

Astringent Herbs (*Stambhana Karma*)

Astringents have a constricting and binding action upon the mucous membranes, organs, skin, and other tissues. They help to prevent the loss of bodily fluids, reduce irritation and inflammation to mucous membranes, and promote the healing of exposed tissues. They pacify both *pitta* and *kapha*, but when used in excess they can increase the dry, rough, and light qualities of *vata*, weakening the digestive fire and causing constipation, gas, muscle spasms, wasting of the tissues, nervousness, and anxiety.

For this reason, care should be taken to choose the proper dosage and duration of treatment. If there is a concern about aggravating *vata*, then combining nutritive tonics along with astringents can be a good approach. It should be noted that all astringent tasting herbs have astringent properties to some extent, but some herbs, such as cayenne, possess astringent properties without having an astringent taste. It is primarily a hot stimulant, but it is also an effective hemostatic herb.

Ayurveda views astringent herbs as having three types of therapeutic actions: Those that are hemostatic (*rakta stambhana*), those that correct excessive discharge of wastes (*mala stambhana*), and those that promote healing of tissues (*ropana*), which are known as vulnerary herbs in Western herbalism. There are astringent herbs that have more than one and sometimes all three therapeutic actions, so further classification (as heating or cooling) may help to understand their energetic differences.

Cooling astringents can be used for bleeding disorders or for stopping diarrhea, especially when due to excess *pitta* in the blood or GI tract. Heating astringent herbs are more specific for *vata* conditions, so when *vata* is involved, especially in the case of diarrhea, heating astringents like *haritaki*, *bilva*, nutmeg, and poppy seeds are useful to bind the stool as well as to help kindle *agni*, promote absorption, and burn *ama*. *Kapha* can benefit from both heating and cooling astringent herbs.

Certain hot pungent herbs like cayenne also have hemostatic properties, but should be avoided or used with caution by *pitta* constitutions or when *pitta* is involved, because they can provoke too much heat in the blood, which may further aggravate the cause of the bleeding if it is related to *pitta* in the first place.

Some astringent herbs are vulnerary and promote the healing of minor cuts, wounds, and burns. Many of these herbs have sweet, demulcent, and emollient properties and make great poultices and pastes for local applications. Not all vulnerary herbs are astringent in action, but they do contain *ropana* properties and help to heal tissues.

Useful vulnerary herbs: Aloe vera, *arjuna*, calendula, chickweed, comfrey, licorice, marshmallow, plantain, self-heal, shepherd's purse, slippery elm, turmeric, witch hazel, and yarrow.

Cooling hemostatic herbs: *Ashoka*, bistort, blackberry, burnet root, cranesbill, goldenseal, hibiscus, horsetail, jasmine, *manjista*, marshmallow, mullein, nettle, oak bark, plantain, pomegranate, saffron, self-heal, shepherd's purse, witch hazel, yarrow, and yellow dock.

Warming pungent hemostatics: Bayberry, cayenne, cinnamon, ginger, *tienchi*, and trillium.

Cooling anti-diarrhea herbs: Alum, apple (stewed), bistort, blackberry, cranesbill, goldenseal, green banana, *kutaja,* lotus seed, meadowsweet, *musta*, oak bark, pearly everlasting, plantain, psyllium, red raspberry, sumach, white pond lily, white rice water, yarrow, and yellow dock.

Hot pungent anti-diarrhea herbs: *Bilva*, black pepper, ginger, *haritaki*, nutmeg, and poppy seeds.

Carminative Herbs (*Vata Anuloman*)

Carminative herbs help to normalize the function and direction of *vata* throughout the entire GI tract, relieving gas and abdominal distention, and normalizing peristaltic movement. They are rich in volatile oils that stimulate *agni*, promote absorption, burn *ama,* increase circulation, and dispel blockages of the bodily channels (*srotamsi*).

Many fragrant culinary spices such as cardamom, coriander, cumin, and ginger are some of our best carminatives and have been used extensively as home remedies as well as in Ayurvedic herbal medicine. Cooking with these herbs helps to make food more digestible. Eating them on a regular basis is a good way to maintain health, prevent disease, and provide the six tastes (*shad rasa*) that play a key role in Ayurvedic nutrition.

Heating carminative herbs are balancing to *kapha* and *vata,* and include *ajwan*, asafoetida, bay leaves, calamus, cardamom, cinnamon, celery seeds, clove, garlic, ginger, nutmeg, oregano, rosemary, thyme, turmeric, and valerian (*tagar*). Heating carminative herbs are primarily pungent in taste and can be quite beneficial to improve the appetite and promote digestion, absorption, and elimination. Pungent is the hottest of the six tastes and is composed of the fire and air elements, so when used in excess it can aggravate *vata*, causing dryness and depletion of the tissues. When used correctly, heating carminatives can counteract the cold quality of *vata*, especially when combined with salt, as in the Ayurvedic digestive formulas *hingwastak churna* and *lavanabhaskar churna*.

Examples of cooling carminative herbs are: Chamomile, coriander, cumin, dill, fennel, *musta* (cypress), peppermint, spearmint, and wintergreen.

Many herbs contain carminative properties, even though they may be better known for other primary actions. Carminatives are often used as assisting herbs to aid in the digestion and absorption of nutritive tonic herbs and herbal compounds in complex formulas.

Demulcent Herbs

Demulcent or emollient herbs are rich in mucilage and are soothing to inflamed and irritated mucous membranes. They typically have a sweet taste and moistening quality, and they pacify both *pitta* and *vata*. Because they are heavy and promote the water element in the body, they tend to increase *kapha* and *ama* when used in excess. They reduce inflammatory conditions throughout the entire GI tract and buffer sensitive tissues from gastric secretions, thus helping to heal gastritis and ulcers. Diarrhea and hyperacidity are often signs of a *pitta* disturbance. Demulcent herbs can be used in those cases to help to absorb the hot, liquid, and spreading qualities of *pitta*.

The benefits of demulcent herbs extend well beyond the GI tract. Herbs such as licorice help to sooth coughs and bronchial irritation, as well as liquefy and expectorate phlegm. Demulcent herbs are also used to treat disorders of the urinary tract. Sometimes referred to as urinary demulcents, they help to ease the pain due to spasms of the bladder and uterus, and can be combined with diuretic herbs to ease the passage of kidney stones.

These types of herbs also have emollient properties and work extremely well in the healing of external wounds and hard-to-heal ulcers. In Ayurveda, herbs that help in the healing of tissues are classified as *ropana*. In Western herbalism, astringent, demulcent, emollient, and vulnerary herbs all have tissue healing properties. Some do because of their soft, oily, or mucilaginous qualities, and others because of their astringency, or even their *prabhava*, or special quality.

Examples of demulcent herbs are: Arrowroot, *bala*, barley, chickweed, coltsfoot, comfrey, corn silk, Irish moss, licorice, *mahabala*, malva, marshmallow, psyllium, *shatavari*, and slippery elm.

Diaphoretic Herbs (*Svedala Karma*)

Diaphoretic herbs induce sweating. They relax and relieve the surface of the body and are used to dispel fever, aching, and chills during acute stages of colds and the flu. In Ayurveda, diaphoretics are classified as having either a warming or cooling action.

Warming diaphoretics purify the plasma and lymphatic tissue, stimulate circulation, remove obstruction of the sweat channels, and eliminate excess *dosha* and impurities through the pores of the skin. They are particularly useful to reduce accumulated cold and wet qualities caused by increased *kapha*, as well as the cold, mobile, or erratic qualities of *vata*. They are primarily pungent like ginger, cinnamon, and *tulsi* and also help to dispel chest and sinus congestion, improve the appetite and digestion, and relieve aching and stiffness due to arthritic complaints.

Cooling diaphoretics pacify the hot, sharp, and spreading qualities of *pitta*. They also balance *kapha*, but can increase *vata* when used in excess. They are typically bitter to pungent in taste, have a cold energy and are effective in clearing heat and bringing down fevers as well as relieving other heat related complaints associated with colds and the flu, such as burning sore throats, swollen glands, cold sores, fever blisters, and headaches. Herbs in this category often possess alterative as well as diuretic properties and also support immunity through the detoxification of the blood.

Examples of warming diaphoretic herbs include: *Ajwan*, black pepper, cayenne, cinnamon, clove, ginger, osha root, rosemary, thyme, sage, and *tulsi*.

Examples of cooling diaphoretics include: Burdock, boneset, blessed thistle, chamomile, coriander, horehound, peppermint, *punarnava*, and yarrow.

Diuretic Herbs (*Mutrala Karma*)

Diuretic herbs help to increase the flow of urine. Their ability to improve the secretion and elimination of the water element, as well as *ama* from the body, extends to all *dhatus* (tissues). They are mainly bitter, astringent, and pungent in taste and pacifying to both *kapha* and *pitta*, because urination is one of the main ways the body releases heat.

Diuretic herbs are used to treat conditions such as water retention, obesity, lymphatic swelling, and urinary or gallstones. Their cooling action helps to relieve damp heat from the kidneys, bladder, liver, and gallbladder. Because most diuretics have a drying action, they may cause constipation, dry skin, and depletion of the tissues, so caution should be used if there is a concern of *vata* aggravation or dehydration, as well as during convalescence. Using strong diuretic herbs in excess for a person who is already in a weakened state, can be likened to whipping a tired horse. However, there are some diuretic herbs that possess moistening and demulcent qualities and even tonic properties, such as *bala*, barley, *gokshura*, and marshmallow.

When using diuretics in a compound, it is always wise to add some soothing demulcent herbs to balance their rough, drying qualities, especially if they are being used to treat urinary stones, in which case demulcents will help to ease the discomfort and facilitate their release.

Cooling diuretic herbs often have diaphoretic, alterative, or antipyretic properties. Some are heating and should be used with care in the case of *pitta* individuals or inflammatory conditions, in which case they can be balanced with cooling herbs.

Some cooling diuretics are: Asparagus, barley, borage, buchu, burdock, cleavers, coriander, corn silk, couch grass, dandelion leaf, fennel, *gokshura*, gravel root, horsetail, lemon grass, marshmallow, nettles, plantain, *punarnava*, *shatavari*, spearmint, and uva ursi.

Some heating diuretics are: *Ajwan*, celery seed, cinnamon, cubebs, juniper berries, Mormon tea, mustard, parsley, pumpkin seeds, and wild carrot.

Emetic Herbs (*Vamana Karma*)

Emetic herbs help to induce vomiting, mainly when given in large doses. In Ayurveda, emetic therapy is called *vamana karma* and is one of the five cleansing measures used in the detoxification program called *Panchakarma*. *Vamana* is primarily used to dispel excess *kapha* and *ama* from the main sites of *kapha* in the upper regions of the body, especially the stomach and respiratory tract. In some situations this therapy can also be used to treat *amla pitta* (sour stomach) and indigestion. Some of the main indications for emetic therapy include sinus problems, repeated fever and flu, respiratory disorders, goiter, diabetes, obesity, food poisoning, lymphatic congestion, skin diseases, epilepsy, fibrocystic changes, and asthma.

In some schools of Western herbalism emetic therapy is also considered a good treatment for asthma, but from an Ayurvedic perspective this may be helpful only for *kapha* types of asthma. This therapy can be dangerous and should only be done under the supervision of a skilled practitioner and according to the individual constitution and *doshic* imbalance.

Emmenagogue Herbs (*Raktabhisarana Karma*)

Emmenagogues are herbs that promote and regulate menstruation. Herbs possessing this action are known in Ayurveda as *raktabhisarana*, or herbs that promote blood flow. They help to increase circulation, remove clotting and congestion, regulate the menstrual cycle, and help with many symptoms relating to the female reproductive system. From an Ayurvedic perspective, they promote the movement of *apana vayu*, the downward moving aspect of *vata* that governs functions such as elimination, menstruation, and ovulation. Because *apana vayu* is responsible for the movement of the fetus during delivery, as a general rule herbs possessing strong emmenagogue properties should not be used during pregnancy because they can stimulate premature labor. Exceptions to this rule are certain mild emmenagogues with rejuvenative properties or herbs such as red raspberry, which are quite safe during pregnancy if used correctly.

To get the best results in treatment, emmenagogues should be chosen according to their energetics. Heating emmenagogues are used for *vata* and *kapha* imbalances of the female reproductive system. *Vata* imbalances can cause delayed menses, cramping, scanty menstrual flow, or amenorrhea. Aggravated *kapha* can cause clotting, water retention, ovarian cysts, and uterine tumors. *Pitta* types of menstrual conditions, such as profuse menstrual flow, vaginal infections, and volatile emotions during menstruation or PMS, are best treated with cooling emmenagogues like aloe vera juice/gel or *manjista*.

Other properties can also be considered when choosing an emmenagogue. For example, some have a diuretic action, like *manjista* and motherwort, and are good for relieving *pitta* and *kapha*. Some are antispasmodic and help with uterine cramping, like black or blue cohosh, cramp bark, *musta*, or valerian. Others are hemostatic and help to prevent excess blood loss, such as *manjista*, rose petals, and yarrow.

In Ayurveda, some emmenagogues are thought to possess tonic properties and act as rejuvenatives to the female reproductive system. These are often sweet, heavy, and moistening. They are beneficial in strengthening and regulating the reproductive organs, building blood, and promoting fertility and longevity. Since there are so many potential causes of menstrual dysfunction, it becomes difficult to attribute any one group of herbs to its treatment. It is best to consider the whole picture of a person to choose the herbs that cover the condition in a holistic manner.

Examples of cooling *raktabhisarana* herbs: Black cohosh, blessed thistle, hibiscus, *manjista*, musta, red raspberry, rose flowers, squaw vine, and yarrow.

Examples of heating *raktabhisarana* herbs: Angelica, asafoetida, cinnamon, ginger, mugwort, myrrh, parsley, pennyroyal, safflower, turmeric, and valerian.

Examples of emmenagogues with rejuvenating properties: Aloe vera, angelica, *ashwagandha*, false unicorn, hibiscus, jasmine, licorice, lotus seeds, myrrh, saffron, *shatavari*, Solomon's seal, *vidari*, and wild yam.

Expectorants (*Kasa Svasahara*)

Expectorants help to expel mucus from the lungs, throat, nasal passages, and stomach. They are effectively used to treat colds, coughs, flu, congestion, and many respiratory disorders. In Sanskrit the term *kasa* refers to "cough" and *svasa* to "difficult breathing." Such disorders are often associated with an imbalance of *kapha dosha*. When *kapha* is increased, it can cause phlegm to accumulate in the stomach and lungs, its primary sites, and from there it can spread throughout the body, clogging and obstructing the *srotas* (bodily channels), and creating abnormal growths such as tumors and cysts.

Heating expectorants are primarily pungent, like ginger or osha, and help to burn and dry up phlegm from the respiratory tract. They also stimulate *agni*, burn *ama*, and are useful for sluggish digestive disorders that can give way to congestive problems.

Cooling expectorants that have a drying or astringent action, like horehound, mullein, or *vamsha rochana*, are indicated for conditions where both *pitta* and *kapha* are involved, which are characterized by yellow to greenish or bloody mucus and sinus pain. Cooling expectorants that are moistening, like licorice or slippery elm, help to liquefy and expel phlegm and soothe inflamed tissues. They are good for treating sore throats and dry coughs and also act as respiratory tonics.

It can often be beneficial to combine expectorants that vary in action to help balance their effects and enhance their overall action. A nice example is the combination of equal parts of ginger and licorice. Ginger helps to balance the heavy, moist qualities of licorice, and licorice helps to counteract the drying and heating qualities of ginger.

Further clarification of symptoms relating to *doshic* involvement can help in choosing the proper expectorant herbs. *Kapha* is the primary *dosha* involved in coughs, colds, and congestive disorders, yet other *doshas* can be present as well. For instance, if *pitta* is aggravated, it can cause symptoms such as yellowish, green, or bloody mucus, sore throat, and a hot feeling in the chest. If *vata* is provoked, there may be symptoms such as thin watery mucus, constricted breathing and wheezing, dry cough, loss of appetite, or chills. There is often more than one *dosha* involved, causing mixed symptoms. In those cases, herbs with varying energies can be used together in formulation.

Some examples of drying expectorants are: Black pepper, boneset, calamus, cardamom, cinnamon, clove, cubebs, elecampane, fenugreek, ginger, horehound, *kantakari*, mustard seeds, orange peel, osha root, *pippali*, sage, *vasaka*, wild ginger, and yerba santa.

Some examples of moistening expectorants are: Chickweed, coltsfoot, comfrey root, fennel, flax seed, Irish moss, licorice, marshmallow, slippery elm, Solomon's seal, sugar, and *vamsha rochana*.

Important cough relieving herbs are: Bayberry, coltsfoot, elecampane, eucalyptus, grindelia, horehound, *kantakari*, licorice, mullein, osha, thyme, *vasaka*, and wild cherry.

Laxatives and Purgatives (*Virechana Karma*)

Laxatives herbs are used to treat constipation, as they help to promote bowel movements and the elimination of *ama* from the intestines. Mild laxatives, also called aperients, are generally slow acting and induce moderate peristalsis. They are mainly moistening and bulking laxatives, like bran, flax seed, licorice, prunes, or psyllium seed, and work well to counter dryness in the colon caused by excess *vata*.

Stronger laxatives are known in Western terminology as purgatives or cathartics, and even stronger ones are called drastics. They work by stimulating the secretion of bile from the gallbladder and activating *samana vayu*, the linear moving *vata* that governs peristalsis. If used improperly or in excess, they can cause diarrhea, griping, tenesmus, and even irritation of the mucous membranes.

Purgatives are typically bitter in taste and have a cooling effect, like mandrake, senna, and rhubarb. Castor oil is also commonly used as a purgative, although it has a heating effect when taken internally. Strong purgative herbs or oils are best taken with carminative herbs like ginger or fennel to ease any discomfort they may cause.

Mild laxatives work well to relieve the occasional bout of constipation, but chronic cases are often difficult to correct and take time and patience. It is important to understand the *doshic* nature and qualities of the condition before choosing the appropriate course of treatment.

Vata related constipation is characterized by dry feces and responds best to moistening laxatives and a *vata* pacifying diet. If the condition becomes chronic it can cause bowel obstruction, so caution should be taken if using purgatives. In such cases, *basti* (herbal enema therapy) can facilitate the breaking up and removal of impacted wastes from the colon before administering the proper laxative.

Even though *pitta* imbalances are typically characterized by loose motion and diarrhea, stagnant *pitta* in the liver and gallbladder can also cause dryness leading to constipation. Here *virechana karma* (purgation) is the best therapy to purge excess heat and bile. Strong or drying laxatives can become irritating to the mucous membrane of the GI tract and should not be used if there is ulcers, gastritis, or colitis.

Kapha types of constipation are characterized by mucus in the stool and accumulated wastes in the colon. Here drying laxatives like *bibhitaki*, *haritaki*, or rhubarb are used to reduce *kapha* and *ama* caused by *manda agni*, or slow digestion.

In some situations, diarrhea that is caused by a build up of toxins in the intestines can be treated briefly with purgative therapy to dispel the toxins causing it. In this case, cooling and bitter purgative herbs are often used.

The Ayurvedic compound *hingwastak* contains various warm pungent herbs and salts that help stimulate the digestive fire and have mild laxative properties, thereby promoting healthy digestion and elimination, and correcting chronic constipation. *Triphala* is a unique compound in that it contains both laxative and tonifying properties and can be used for extended periods of time to detoxify, regulate bowel function, and rejuvenate the body.

Laxative herbs should be used with care and with a holistic approach to avoid further weakening the bowel tone and causing dependency. Women should not use strong laxatives during pregnancy so as not to over stimulate *apana vayu*, the downward moving aspect of *vata*, because this can cause premature labor. Here fiber rich foods and soaked fruits such as prunes, dates, and raisins are better choices.

Examples of bulking and moistening laxatives: Bran, castor oil, dates, flax seed, *ghee*, licorice, marshmallow, prunes, psyllium husk, raisins, salt, *shatavari*, and warm milk.

Examples of strong laxatives or purgatives: Castor oil, croton, epsom salt, *haritaki*, *indravaruni kumari* (aloe vera powder), mandrake, rhubarb, and senna.

Examples of cooling laxatives: Aloe vera, blue flag, cascara sagrada, *kutki*, rhubarb, senna, *trivrit*, and yellow dock.

Lithotriptic (Anti-Lithic) Herbs

These are herbs that help to dissolve and eliminate stones of the gallbladder, kidneys, and urinary tract. In Ayurveda, these herbs fall under the category of herbs with *bhedaniya* (breaking) action to accumulations caused by excess *kapha*. Many of these herbs also have diuretic action such as *pashana bheda* and *gokshura*, as well as Western herbs like cleavers, dandelion, gravel root, and parsley.

Lithotriptic herbs such as cascara sagrada, *kutki*, and Oregon grape root have an affinity to the gallbladder and act as cholagogues, helping to purge excess heat and bile from the gallbladder.

> **Examples of lithotriptics:** *Ajwan*, buchu leaf, cleavers, corn silk, cranberry, dandelion, *gokshura*, gravel root, horsetail, juniper berries, *kutki*, *manjista*, Oregon grape root, *pashanabheda*, and uva ursi.

Nervines

Herbs with nervine properties help to support the nervous system. Many of these herbs are aromatic and help to enhance the flow of *prana*, the vital energy or intelligence responsible for all functions within the body, from the grossest to the subtlest levels. Nervines are calming and refreshing to the mind, increase awareness, and enliven the senses. In Ayurveda, a similar category of herbs that strengthen mental function are referred to as *medhya rasayanas*. Many nervines, such as gotu kola, skullcap, *jatamansi*, and calamus, fall into this class of herbs.

Some nervines have sedative or relaxant properties and can calm and replenish the nervous system when over stimulated from general stress, emotional imbalances, or excessive work. They ground the light and mobile qualities of *vata* and can be used to treat a wide variety of *vata* disorders, such as anxiety, nervousness, insomnia, numbness, sciatica, joint and muscle pain, and neurological diseases. Many nervine sedatives are also antispasmodic and help to relieve cramping, muscle spasms, coughs, asthma, tics, tremors, epilepsy, and convulsions.

Other nervines are stimulants and help to clear obstructions of the nerve channels (*majjavaha srotas*). They are particularly useful when excess *kapha* and *ama* block the normal movement of *vata*. Certain nourishing tonic herbs also have nervine properties. They are valuable for nourishing and strengthening the nerve tissue and are particularly useful in deficient conditions. One such herb is *ashwagandha*, which is one of the best rejuvenating tonics (*rasayanas*) for *vata*.

Nervines can also be categorized as either heating or cooling. Heating nervines, like calamus, balance *vata* and *kapha*. Cooling nervines, such as gotu kola, *jatamansi*, or skullcap, help to pacify *pitta*. Heating sedative herbs, like valerian, are often used to treat hypermobile, *vata* related disorders of the mind and nervous system, whereas warming and stimulating herbs like calamus and sage may be more beneficial to treat obstructed *vata*.

Cooling nervines often have blood cleansing properties as well, and help to calm the hot headed nature of *pitta* by clearing heat from the blood, liver, and nervous system. Those with a bitter taste usually have a drying quality and help to relieve *kapha*. Some, like gotu kola and *jatamansi*, are considered *tridoshic*.

As usual, many nervine herbs have other properties too, and should be selected according to the individual case. Some nervines are also carminatives and can help to kindle *agni*, burn *ama*, and relieve flatulence and abdominal discomfort. Others have bronchial dilating properties to help relieve spasms of the bronchial tubes, and can be effective for treating respiratory tract disorders such as asthma and bronchitis.

> **Examples of heating nervine and antispasmodic herbs are:** Asafoetida, *ashwagandha*, basil, bayberry, calamus, camphor, cramp bark, eucalyptus, garlic, *guggulu*, lady's slipper, mugwort, myrrh, nutmeg, pennyroyal, poppy seeds, sage, *tulsi*, and valerian.

> **Examples of cooling nervines and antispasmodic herbs are:** Betony, *bhringaraj*, black haw, catnip, chamomile, gotu kola, hops, jasmine, *jatamansi*, lavender, lemon balm, motherwort, mullein, oat straw, passion flower, peppermint, sandalwood, skullcap, St. John's wort, vervain, *vidari*, and wild yam.

Nutritive Tonics (*Bruhana Karma*)

Nutritive tonic herbs build and strengthen the tissues and increase body weight. They are typically sweet in taste and post-digestive effect, and have heavy, moist, oily, and softening qualities. In general, they are more pacifying to *pitta* and *vata* but may increase *kapha* and *ama*, especially when taken by those with poor digestion or high *ama* conditions.

They are best used in *nirama* conditions (that is, when *ama* is not combined with the *dosha*) or along with pungent and carminative herbs like ginger or cardamom to promote their digestion and absorption. When *ama* is combined with the *dosha* (*sama dosha*), emphasis should be placed on detoxification first.

Traditionally, nutritive tonics are mixed with other nutritive substances like milk, *ghee*, honey, and raw sugar to enhance their rejuvenating effects. Even though in excess they tend to increase *kapha*, nutritive tonics like licorice or marshmallow root can help to liquefy and expectorate *kapha* in the form of phlegm. For this purpose, they combine well with warm, spicy herbs like ginger, wild ginger, or *pippali* to balance and support their decongesting and expectorating action.

Nutritive herbs with a bitter taste and cooling energy like comfrey root, *shatavari*, *vidari*, or wild yam are great for pacifying *pitta* and may also be used for treating *vata* related conditions, especially when a bitter herb is needed but without being depleting to the body as stronger bitter herbs tend to be.

Warming nutritive tonics like *ashwagandha* and ginseng are the best tonics for *vata* and are often indicated when there is general weakness or fatigue. Such herbs can be helpful in a wide variety of deficient types of diseases. They are extremely beneficial for those in their *vata* years of life (over 50 years of age) to promote strength, vitality, and longevity.

Many demulcent herbs are also categorized as nutritive tonics. Being rich in mucilage, they work well in treating *pitta* related condition of the GI tract, and help to protect, soothe, and heal irritated mucous membranes. They also increase the water element in the body and counter dryness caused by excess *vata*.

> **Examples of nutritive tonics are:** Almonds, *amalaki*, angelica, apricots, *bala*, blue green algae, cashews, coconut, comfrey root, *dashamula*, dates, date sugar, flax seed, *ghee*, Irish moss, jaggary, kapi kacchu, kelp, licorice, lotus seed, marshmallow, milk, raisins, raw honey, rehmannia, saw palmetto, seaweed, *shatavari*, slippery elm, Solomon's seal, sugar cane, *vidari*, and wild yam.

Rejuvenative Tonics (*Rasayana Karma*)

Unique to Ayurveda, *rasayanas* are considered to be the most effective group of herbs for rejuvenation. *Rasayana* literally means "to enter the *rasa*," the water element of the body (plasma and lymph) with which all tissues are bathed and nourished. *Rasayanas* help to kindle the *agni* present within all the *dhatus* and ensure optimal tissue development, as well as the final formation of *ojas*, the vital essence of all bodily tissues. They promote the regeneration and revitalization of all cells, tissues, and organs, and increase immunity, vitality, mental function, and longevity.

Much like nutritive tonics, *rasayanas* are often sweet in taste and *vipak* (post-digestive effect). They often possess heavy, oily, and moistening qualities and are pacifying to both *vata* and *pitta*. Some *rasayanas* are pungent in taste with a warming energy and are more beneficial for *kapha* and *vata*, while others are cooling and more pacifying to *pitta*. It should be noted that some herbs and compounds are considered *rasayanas* because of the dramatic effect they have on a particular tissue or organ.

Rasayanas act primarily through their *prabhava*, or special potency, which cannot always be explained with the Ayurvedic theory of taste, energy, post-digestive effect, or even by modern biochemistry. Nevertheless, their benefits on the body, mind, and consciousness have been observed by Ayurvedic physicians for thousands of years.

The ancient texts state that in order to receive the optimum benefits from *rasayana* therapy, one must first undergo proper cleansing therapies such as *Panchakarma* to remove *ama*. After deep cleansing, *rasayanas* can act without obstruction, working down to the cellular level, and have the ability to bestow youthfulness, luster, strength, intelligence, and longevity.

Spiritual practices such as mantra, prayer, ritual, yogic disciplines, spiritual self-inquiry, and meditation have profound rejuvenating effects upon the body and consciousness, and can be considered *rasayanas* as well.

Examples of *vata rasayanas*: *Ashwagandha*, bala, calamus, *dashamula*, fo-ti, garlic, *ghee*, ginseng, *guggulu*, *haritaki*, jaggary, kapi kacchu, licorice, onion, saw palmetto, sesame seeds, sugar, *vidari*, and warm milk.

Examples of *pitta rasayanas*: Aloe vera gel/juice, *amalaki*, *bala*, *brahmi* (or gotu kola), comfrey root, fo-ti, *ghee*, ginger, *gokshura*, *guduchi*, licorice, *manjista*, milk, rock candy, saffron, *shatavari*, and *vidari*.

Examples of *kapha rasayanas*: *Bibhitaki*, elecampane (*pushkaramula*), *guggulu*, honey, *pippali*, and *shilajit*.

Stimulant and Digestive Herbs (*Dipana-Pachana Karma*)

Stimulant herbs invigorate the body and enhance its functions. In Ayurveda stimulants are classified as *agni dipana*, or herbs that kindle the digestive fire (*jathara agni*), and *ama pachana*, or herbs that burn *ama* by stimulating *jathara agni* and *pachak pitta* present in the stomach and small intestine. Many culinary spices fall into this category of herbs and are used in cooking to enhance the flavor and help in the digestion of rich and heavy foods, as well as to reduce the *vata* provoking qualities of foods such as potatoes, cabbage, beans, or broccoli. They are typically heating, pacify to *kapha* and *vata*, and regulate *samana vayu,* the subtype of *vata* responsible for digestion, absorption, and assimilation.

Due to their hot energy, stimulants can increase *pitta* and cause dryness, which can provoke *vata* when taken in excess. They are indicated where there is an increase of *dosha* or *ama* and can even be used in moderation in *sama pitta* conditions. They are often combined with bitter herbs like barberry, *guduchi,* or *amalaki* to balance their heating effects.

Stimulant herbs promote circulation, break up obstructions in the channels, and help to prevent diseases caused by the accumulation of *ama*. They often possess diaphoretic, expectorant, antiseptic, and carminative properties as well. They can be used to bring down superficial types of fevers by burning the *ama* causing them and promoting sweating.

> **Examples of stimulant herbs are:** *Ajwan*, asafoetida, black pepper, cardamom, cayenne, clove, fenugreek, garlic, ginger, horseradish, mustard seeds, onion, *pippali*, and prickly ash.

Cooling stimulants, which are *pitta* pacifying, can be found in the bitter tonic category and are recommended for short-term use. Ayurveda views bitter taste as being cold, so it will eventually weaken the *agni*. Peppermint is one of the best cooling stimulants and can be combined with equal parts ginger, cumin seeds, and fennel to make a *pitta* pacifying digestive tea.

Ayurvedic Classification of Therapeutic Actions

In the classical Ayurvedic texts herbs are classified according to their specific therapeutic actions. Below is a brief table of these categories with several examples of Eastern and Western herbs and substances that relate to them.

Actions	Functions	Substances
Anulomana: Carminative	Expel gas and waste products, promote proper digestion, absorption and assimilation	*Ajwan*, asafoetida, coriander, cumin, fennel, ginger, *haritaki*, parsley, peppermint, rock salt
Arshoghna: Anti-hemorrhoidal	Help relieve and heal hemorrhoids	Aloe vera, calamus, castor oil, coconut oil, goldenseal, *guduchi*, *hari-taki*, *kama dudha*, *kutaja*, milk thistle, *nagkeshar*, *neem*, ocotillo, Oregon grape root, rasp-berry leaf, turmeric
Artala: Enhancing the ovum	Enhance the health of the ovum	Aloe vera, evening primrose oil, licorice, *shatavari*, soy, *vidari*, wild yam
Balya: Tonifying	Promote strength	*Ashwagandha*, *bala*, dates soaked in *ghee*, ginseng, *shatavari*, *vidari*
Bhedaniya: Breaking down of accumulations	Break down of hard accumulations like old impacted wastes, gallstones and kidney stones	*Ajwan*, castor oil, *chitrak*, dandelion, gravel root, *kutki*, *kutaja*, *pashan bheda*, senna

Actions	Functions	Substances
Bruhaniya: Anabolic or bulking	Increase weight and promote the growth of bodily tissues	Almonds, *amalaki*, apricots, *ashwagandha*, *bala*, cashews, coconut, *dashamula*, *kapi kacchu*, marshmallow, *shatavari*, *vidari*
Dahaprashamana: Heat relieving	Relieve burning sensations on the skin	*Kama dudha*, guduchi, *gulwel sattva*, lotus leaf, raw sugar, rose, sandalwood, *shanka bhasma*, *shatavari*, turmeric, vetivert
Dipaniya/ Pachaniya: Digestive stimulant	Kindle the digestive fire (*agni*) and burn *ama*	*Ajwan*, asafoetida, black pepper, cardamom, *chitrak*, cinnamon, clove, ginger, *pippali*, rock salt
Hridya: Heart tonifying	Strengthen heart function.	*Arjuna*, *ashwagandha*, elecampane (*pushkaramula*), garlic, hawthorne berries, mistle toe, motherwort, pomegranate fruit, *rudraksha*, *sarpagandha*, *shringa bhasma*

Actions	Functions	Substances
Jivaniya: Vitalizing	Help to support life energy and promote longevity	Blue green algae, ginseng, Irish moss, licorice, mung beans, *sanjivani*, sesame seeds, *urud dal*, *vidari*
Jwarahara: Febrifuge or antipyretic	Lower fevers	Boneset, *guduchi*, *mahasudarshan*, *manjista*, *swedala* herbs, *tulsi*, yarrow
Kandughna: Anti-pruritic	Relieve itching	Barberry, licorice, *manjista*, *neem*, turmeric
Kanthya: Nourishing to the throat	Soothe sore throat and improve the voice	Bayberry, camphor, cardamom, cinnamon, clove, ginger, *haritaki*, licorice, marshmallow, raisins, rock candy, slippery elm, *vidari*
Kasahara: Cough suppressant	Anti-tussive, anti-spasmodic	Coltfoot, *haritaki*, *kantakari*, osha, *punarnava*, raisins, *sitopaladi*, *talisadi*, *shringa bhasma*, *vasa*, wild cherry bark
Keshyam: Promoting hair growth	Strengthen hair roots and prevent graying and premature loss	*Amalaki*, *bhringaraj*, *brahmi*, *dashamula*, hibiscus, licorice, nettles, rosemary, sage, skullcap

Actions	Functions	Substances
Krimighna: Anthelmintic	Destroy parasites	Asafoetida, betel nut, black walnut, grapefruit seed extract, *kutaja*, *neem*, pumpkin seeds, *shardunika*, *vidanga*, wormwood
Lekaniya: Reducing	Scrape fat and reduce excess *kapha* and accumulations.	Black pepper, barberry, calamus (*vacha*), *chitrak*, copper *bhasma* or water, honey, hot water, *kutki*, *musta* (cypress), *shilajit*, turmeric
Mutrala: Diuretic	Promote urination	Asparagus, cleavers, coriander, dandelion leaf, *gokshura*, gravel root, juniper berries, *kamala*, *punarnava*
Nirajanana: Nervine sedative	Calm the nervous system	*Ashwagandha*, chamomile, garlic, hops, kava kava, nutmeg, skullcap, *tagar*, valerian
Rasayana: Rejuvenating	Slow aging, nourish and rejuvenate tissues	*Amalaki*, apricot, *ashwagandha*, *bibhitaki*, comfrey root, *gulwel sattva*, *haritaki*, licorice, *pippali*, *shatavari*, *vidari*, wild yam

Actions	Functions	Substances
***Samjna-Sthapana*:** Restoring consciousness	Restore consciousness as from coma or delirium	Asafoetida, calamus (*vacha*), camphor, *brahmi*, *jatamansi*, *jyotishmati*, onion juice, skullcap
***Sandhaniya*:** Joining or healing of tissues	Promote healing of cuts, wounds, ulcers, bones, ligaments and tendons	Aloe vera, *arjuna*, bayberry, comfrey leaf, *guggulu*, *gulwel sattva*, licorice, licorice *ghee*, *manjista*, plantain, turmeric
***Shitaprashamana*:** Relieving cold	Relieve cold sensations on the skin	*Agaru*, black pepper, calamus (*vacha*), cayenne, cinnamon, ginger, hawthorne berry, *pippali*, prickly ash, valerian
***Shotahara*:** Diuretic and astringent	Relieve edema and swelling	*Bilva*, cleavers, dandelion, *gokshura*, *manjista*, *punarnava*
***Shukrala*:** Promoting growth of sperm	Increase sperm count	*Ashwagandha*, garlic, ginseng, kapi kacchu, licorice, lotus root, milk, onion, *shilajit*, *urud dal*

Actions	Functions	Substances
Shula-Prashamana: Relieving colic	Relieve intestinal cramping	*Ajwan*, asafoetida, chamomile, cardamom, catnip, cumin, dill, fennel, ginger, *pippali*, rock salt
Smriti Vardhak: Enhancing memory	Improve mental functions and memory	*Ashwagandha*, *brahmi*, calamus (*vacha*), ginkgo biloba, *jyotishmati*, *shankapushpi*
Svedala: Diaphoretic, promoting sweating	Dilate the pores of the skin	Cardamom, cinnamon, ginger, lemon grass, *musta*, tulsi, yarrow
Swasahara: Relieving asthma	Open bronchi and ease breathing	*Abrak bhasma*, cardamom, elecampane (*pushkaramula*), ephedra, *kantakari*, licorice, lobelia, mullein, osha, *pippali*, *punarnava*, *tulsi*, *vasa*, *vamsha rochana*
Vajikarana: Aphrodisiac	Enhance reproductive organs and tissues	Angelica, *ashwagandha*, kapi kacchu, milk, *shatavari*, Solomon's seal, *vidari*, wild yam

Actions	Functions	Substances
Vamaka: Emetic	Induce vomiting	Calamus (*vacha*), cardamom, licorice, lobelia, *madanphala* (nux vomica), *neem*, salt, *vidanga*
Varnya: Enhancing complexion	Improve the luster and tone of the skin	Calendula, lavender, lotus root, *manjista*, rose, sandalwood, turmeric
Virechana: Purgative	Strong laxative	Cascara sagrada, castor oil, chamomile, *haritaki*, *kutki*, rhubarb, senna, *trivrit*

Ayurvedic Herbal Energetic Concepts

A unique aspect of Ayurvedic herbology is its energetic model, which classifies herbs and other medicinal substances according to their *rasa* (taste), *virya* (energy or strength), *vipak* (post-digestive effect) and *prabhava* (unique or special potency). This practical system provides the herbalist with a theoretical basis for understanding how a substance affects the body, as well as how to make the most appropriate choices of herbal medicines for each particular situation.

Knowledge of the *rasa, virya*, and *vipak* of herbs can help the herbalist to perceive them in a holistic manner and understand how their qualities relate to the qualities and *doshas* involved in each individual case, as well as their immediate actions and long-term effects. Therefore, these basic Ayurvedic concepts can be an invaluable tool to broaden the knowledge of all medicinal plants the world over, so as to use and combine them with a more holistic, constitutional approach.

Rasa: Taste

The Sanskrit word *rasa* has many meanings. The taste of any substance is experienced through the presence of the water element (saliva) on the tongue. So *rasa,* aside from meaning taste, also means the "juice" or "sap" of plants, as well as the lymph and plasma of our bodies (as in *rasa dhatu*). *Rasa* is also suggestive of the enthusiasm, appreciation, and liveliness that are the result of a harmonious balance of the six tastes (*shad raśa*) on the tongue and in the body.

Ayurveda places great emphasis upon the knowledge of these six tastes in herbs, food, and culinary spices, as well as their effects on the body, mind, and consciousness. When herbs are tasted directly on the tongue, their *rasa* is quickly perceived and conveyed to the entire organism through the nervous system (via the *prana*, or flow of intelligence). For this reason, Ayurveda recommends that, whenever possible, herbs should be tasted. Powdered formulas can be taken in tea form and tablets chewed to some degree to release their taste on the tongue. It can be said that the medicinal effect of any substance begins with its initial taste.

A balance of the six tastes is vital to the health of *agni*, the digestive fire, and the absorption and assimilation of nutrients. Certain tastes have an affinity to specific organs and a direct effect on our thoughts, feelings, and emotions. A good example of this is in the sense of contentment and satisfaction that we have after eating a well spiced meal that contains a balanced blend of *shad rasa*. If any of the six tastes is missing or taken in excess in our daily diet, we may feel that our food does not digest well or that we are lacking something, which often manifests as excessive or unhealthy cravings.

Virya: Energy

Virya means energy, strength, power, or potency. It is the basic action of a substance that affects *jathara agni*, the central digestive fire, as well as all the *dhatu agnis*, or digestive components of each tissue. It has an immediate effect on the body. **There are eight qualities of *virya* (known as *ashtavidha virya*)**: Hot, cold, heavy, light, soft, sharp, oily, and dry. Out of these eight types, the heating and cooling qualities have the most direct effect upon the *agni* and the metabolism, while the others are subtler and can only be perceived over time.

Substances possessing a heating *virya* are primarily pacifying to *vata* and *kapha*. They kindle the digestive fire, burn *ama*, increase body temperature, and promote circulation. When used in excess, or for extended periods, they can diminish *ojas* and provoke *pitta*, thus causing hyperactive metabolism, catabolic activity (destruction), hypoglycemia, bleeding, ulcers, and many inflammatory conditions.

Substances possessing a cooling *virya* pacify *pitta* and increase *kapha* and *vata*. They promote anabolic activity (growth), relieve burning and inflammation, and decrease body temperature. When used in excess, they can suppress *agni*, thus weakening the power of digestion and causing malabsorption and *ama* formation.

Sweet is the least cooling of all tastes. There are some sweet substances that are exceptions to this rule, like honey, molasses, and jaggary, which are sweet but have a heating effect due to their *prabhava*, or special potency.

Sour taste is heating, with the exception of certain sour substances such as limes (in moderation) and *amalaki* fruit, which are *pitta* pacifying despite their sour taste.

Salty taste is heating, which can be easily inferred by the burning effect salt has when applied to an open wound.

Pungent is the hottest of all six tastes, as can be experienced when biting into a chili, a clove, or raw garlic.

Bitter is the most cooling taste and is present in herbs like dandelion, goldenseal, and *neem*, all of which have a strong *pitta* pacifying effect on the body.

Astringent taste is cooling. It is constricting and healing to the tissues and membranes, and is present in herbs like alum, *ashoka*, *manjista*, plantain, red raspberry, white oak bark, and witch hazel.

Vipak: Post-Digestive Effect

There are six stages of digestion. Throughout these stages, the taste of food is also transformed. As it moves through the GI tract, it goes through the sweet, sour, salty, pungent, bitter, and astringent phases. *Vipak* (also *vipaka*), or post-digestive effect, is the final stage in the transformation of taste. It takes place in the colon, where the six tastes are then reduced to sweet, sour, or pungent. Sweet and salty tastes have sweet *vipak*; sour taste has sour *vipak*; and bitter, pungent, and astringent tastes yield a pungent *vipak*. *Vipak* is present in the waste products (urine, feces, and sweat) and plays a role in the absorption of nutrients and the elimination process. The properties of *vipak* are similar to those of *rasa*, but *vipak* is slower to show its effects.

Sweet *vipak* is anabolic and builds *kapha*. It increases the water element, thus promoting the elimination of urine, feces, and sweat.

Sour *vipak* promotes metabolic activity and helps to kindle *agni*, but in excess it can aggravate *pitta*, causing acidic pH, loose stools, or diarrhea.

Pungent *vipak* has a stimulating and catabolic action. In excess, it tends to aggravate *vata* and in time may also increase *pitta*, causing constipation, flatulence, and painful urination. Pungent *vipak* also has more specific effects depending on whether it comes from pungent, bitter, or astringent tastes. Pungent *vipak* derived from pungent substances may cause imbalances such as skin conditions that are dry and irritating, hemorrhoids, and irritable bowel. Pungent *vipak* from bitter *rasa* is more cooling and can cause low libido and diminish the sperm count. Pungent *vipak* from astringent taste is more likely to produce ailments such as joint pain, fissures, fistula, and osteoporosis.

The knowledge of *vipak* provides another useful tool to determine the overall effect a substance may have over the course of time and to avoid imbalances caused by the long-term use of certain herbs and foods.

Prabhava: Special Action

As much as Ayurveda places great emphasis on the energetic model of *rasa*, *virya*, and *vipak*, it also takes into account what is known as *prabhava*, which is a special and unique action or potency that certain substances may possess. *Prabhava* is an action that cannot be explained by the Ayurvedic energetic model or by any materialistic or biochemical viewpoint. It can only be understood as the special potency of a plant or substance that can affect the body and mind on a direct and subtle levels. It goes beyond the realm of herbs and is, in essence, the unexplainable power within creation. This unique action can be perceived in various ways, such as the effects that sound, color, and nature have upon our state of mind, the power of mantras and rituals, or the influence of planets on our individual lives. Despite our technological advancements in science, much is still not understood so as to explain the dynamic and profound effects that herbs can have upon the body, mind, and consciousness.

Sometimes two herbs have the same *rasa*, *virya*, and *vipak* and yet remarkably different actions. This is viewed as *prabhava*. Furthermore, depending upon the dosage given, a substance can have the exact opposite of its expected effect, and this is also *prabhava*. For instance, *ghee* in small amounts can help to bind the stool, where as large amounts have a laxative effect. Another example of *prabhava* can be seen with herbs like turmeric, barberry, or *guduchi* , all of which have a powerful cooling and anti-inflammatory effect despite their heating *virya*. Likewise, even though sweet taste is cooling and increases *kapha*, honey, which is most definitely sweet, is heating and helps to decrease *kapha*.

Since time immemorial, Ayurveda has embraced the study and observation of the unexplainable, adding it to its wealth of valuable knowledge of foods and medicines. Native American and many other indigenous cultures also honor this mystical side of things, but much of this knowledge has become obscured in our modern, overly scientific world. Yet through our keen observation, such exploration into the spiritual, mystical, and unexplainable can greatly benefit the path of herbalism in the West. (See chart on *Rasa*, *Virya*, and *Vipak*.)

Shad Rasa: Six Tastes

Ayurveda detects six tastes: Sweet, sour, salty, pungent, bitter, and astringent. Each of these tastes is made up primarily of two elements but contains all five to some degree. Sweet taste is mainly composed of earth and water; sour taste of fire and earth; salty taste of fire and water; pungent taste of fire and air; bitter taste of air and ether; and astringent taste of earth and air.

Sweet Taste (*Madhura Rasa*)

Sweet taste is the first taste to touch the tongue as we nurse at our mother's breast. It brings contentment and pleasure to the mind and sense organs. Sweet taste is made up primarily of the earth and water elements, and possesses cooling, heavy, and oily qualities, as well as anabolic, demulcent, and emollient properties. It is nourishing and strengthening to all the tissues, and is valuable for young children or for those who are emaciated, aged, or recovering from a serious illness.

Sweet increases *ojas*, the essence of all bodily tissues, and promotes longevity. It improves the voice and relieves thirst and burning sensations. In the classical texts it is recommended to make rejuvenating herbal preparations with sweet substances like raw sugar, milk, and clarified butter. This is considered the best way to rejuvenate the system after detoxification has taken place. An example of this is the herbal jam *Chyavanprash*.

Excess sweet taste is mainly associated with *kapha* disorders, but it can affect any of the *doshas*. It can weaken the digestion, causing loss of appetite, repeated colds, congestion, lethargy, obesity, edema, and diabetes, as well as abnormal growths like tumors (usually benign) and cysts.

Sweet taste is present in all sugars and starches, as well as in foods like milk, rice, almonds, sweet fruits, and wheat. Many sweet herbs are pleasant to the taste. Some examples are: Fennel, flax seed, licorice, marshmallow, *shatavari*, slippery elm, *vidari*, and wild yam.

Sour Taste (*Amla Rasa*)

Sour taste is made up of the fire and earth elements and is hot, light, sharp, acidic, moistening, and nourishing. It is pacifying to *vata* but increases *pitta*. In excess, it provokes *kapha*, but in small amounts it can increase the metabolism and burn fat and *ama*. Sour increases salivary secretions and stimulates the digestive fire and the appetite.

Sour is refreshing and encourages elimination. It is antispasmodic and helps to correct the movement of *vata*, relieving gas, bloating, and abdominal discomfort. Sour herbs like *amalaki* and hawthorne berry are also good for the heart.

In excess, sour taste can cause looseness of the body, loss of strength, sensitivity of the teeth, skin diseases, toxic blood, itching, thirst, and burning of the stomach, throat, chest, heart, and urethra. It can also contribute to diarrhea, edema, jaundice, fever, dysentery, and respiratory congestion.

> **Examples of herbs and fruits with sour taste are:** *Amalaki*, hawthorne berries, lemons, limes, rose hips, and sour berries.

Salty Taste (*Lavana Rasa*)

Salty taste is made up of the fire and water elements. It pacifies *vata* and provokes *pitta* and *kapha* in excess. It is hot, sharp, heavy, and oily, and promotes water retention. It decreases muscular rigidity, creates electrolyte balance, and clears obstructed channels and pores by liquefying *kapha*. It also increases salivation, causes sweating, kindles the digestive fire, and promotes elimination, but in large doses it can have an emetic effect and induce vomiting.

When taken in excess, salty taste can cause ailments such as blood stagnation, hypertension, skin conditions, gout, premature hair loss, wrinkling of the skin, edema, herpes, impotence, bleeding disorders, and hyperacidity.

There are very few herbs with a salty taste, although in Ayurvedic medicine adding certain types of salt to herbal formulas is quite common and can be seen in such compounds as *hingwastak churna, lavanabhaskar churna*, or *chitrakadi bati*. Eating mineral rich sea vegetables like kelp, nori, and kombu is one of the healthiest ways to obtain salty taste from the plant kingdom.

Pungent Taste (*Katu Rasa*)

Pungent taste is made up of the fire and air elements and has light, dry, and heating qualities. It pacifies *kapha* but aggravates *pitta*. In small amounts, the hot nature of pungent taste helps to calm *vata*, but in excess it can increase its light and dry qualities. It improves the circulation, stimulates the appetite, and promotes digestion and absorption. It is a natural expectorant that encourages nasal secretions, sweat, and tears, and also burns fat.

Pungent taste can help break up hard masses, aid in the elimination of waste products, and rid the body of *ama*, germs, parasites, and worms. It is useful in the treatment of edema, obesity, skin growths, and blood stagnation, as well as clotting.

Overuse of pungent taste can cause thirst, hiccup, choking, depletion of the reproductive tissues, fatigue, and fainting. Due to its *pitta* provoking action, it can create burning sensations, diarrhea, heartburn, and nausea. Pungent taste is often referred to as acrid, spicy, or aromatic.

> **Common pungent herbs include:** angelica, anise, asafoetida (*hing*), bayberry, bay leaves, black pepper, cardamom, cayenne, cinnamon, clove, coriander, cumin, fennel, garlic, ginger, horse radish, mustard seeds, peppermint, *pippali*, prickly ash, rosemary, sage, thyme, and valerian.

Bitter Taste (*Tikta Rasa*)

Bitter contains the air and ether elements, and its qualities are light, dry, and cool. It mitigates *pitta* and *kapha*, relieving burning sensations and fever. In moderation, it stimulates digestion, improves the appetite, and cleanses the intestines of *ama* and parasites. It purifies the blood and is useful in treating skin diseases like eczema, psoriasis, and leprosy.

Excess bitter taste increases the dry and light qualities of *vata* and can cause depletion of the muscle, fat, bone marrow, and reproductive tissues.

> **Some common bitter herbs are:** barberry, *bhringaraj*, burdock (seeds and root), chicory, dandelion, echinacea, eyebright, gentian, goldenseal, gotu kola, *kutki*, *neem*, Oregon grape, pau d'arco, rhubarb, yarrow, and yellow dock.

Astringent Taste (*Kasaya Rasa*)

The earth and air elements make up the astringent taste. It increases *vata* and decreases both *kapha* and *pitta*. It has cool, dry, and light qualities. It relieves digestive disorders and inflamed mucous membranes, and binds the stool. It dries moisture, tightens tissues, and helps to stop bleeding and profuse sweating. It also heals ulcers, wounds, and gum disease, and knits broken bones. Its drying action helps to reduce fat tissue and is used to treat obesity.

When used in excess, astringent taste can cause constipation, obstructions, flatulence, weak digestion, and malabsorption. It also causes drying of the skin, excessive thirst, emaciation, nervous disorders, and loss of virility.

As a general rule, astringents, especially strong ones, should not be taken for extended periods due to their depleting effect on the tissues and digestive system.

> **Some common astringent herbs are:** American cranesbill, *ashoka*, *bilva*, goldenseal, horsetail, lotus seed, meadowsweet, oak bark, plantain, pomegranate, raspberry leaves, sage, shepherd's purse, sumach, uva ursi, *vamsha rochana*, white pond lily, witch hazel, and yarrow.

Psychological Actions of the Six Tastes

Sweet taste is often associated with a feeling of love and contentment. If there is an imbalance of sweet taste, or a lack of contentment, one may seek fulfillment through indulging in sweet foods. Sweet taste brings positive memories, thoughts of loved ones and feelings of devotion. Sweet foods are often used in India as symbolic offerings of love (*prasadam*) to a deity or guru. Likewise, in the West, chocolates and candy are given to loved ones as a token of friendship and appreciation. Even when we express our affection we use words like "sweetie," "honey," and so on. Yet too much sweet taste creates greed, attachment, and complacency.

Sour taste is hot and sharp, and therefore aids with concentration, sharpening the intellect, and increasing awareness. An imbalance of sour taste can cause feelings of anger, envy, and criticism, which may be the result of unfulfilled desires. Interestingly enough, someone who complains a lot, is peevish or grumpy is often referred to as a "sour apple" or a "sour puss."

Just as salt enhances the flavor of foods, salty taste lifts the spirit and sparks interest in life. Like sweet taste, it increases *kapha* when used in excess and is associated with emotions like possessiveness, greed, and attachment. Indulgence in salty taste promotes temptation, desires, and addictions.

Pungent taste is associated with the drive and motivation of *pitta* types and brings enthusiasm, vigor, and vitality. It improves concentration and sharpens the mind and intellect. In excess, it can provoke *pitta*, promoting feelings of anger, irritability, jealousy, and aggressiveness.

Bitter taste creates aversion to desires, aiding in celibacy, and promotes introversion and introspection. In excess, it will make a person dissatisfied, cynical, and boring, and may create isolation and loneliness as a result.

Astringent taste, due to its earth element, is supporting and grounding, and helps to bring together scattered thoughts, feelings, and emotions. In excess, it aggravates *vata*, leading to fear, anxiety, restlessness, depression, and absentmindedness.

Herbal Preparations and Therapeutics

The Five Main Plant Preparations (*Pancha Kasaya Kalpana*)

In Ayurveda there are five main preparations of raw plants to be used as medicine: The freshly expressed juice of the plant (*swarasa*); the pulp or paste (*kalka*); the decoction (*kvatha*); a hot infusion (*phanta*); and a cold infusion (*hima* or *sita kasaya*). They are listed below in order of strength, from strongest to weakest.

Fresh Juice (*Swarasa*)

The fresh juice of the raw plant can be obtained by crushing or pounding it with a large mortar and pestle or grinding stone. It is then pressed and strained through a clean cloth. A wheat grass or Champion juicer can also work well for some juicy plants. Sometimes, as in the case of plants with hard leaves or stems, crushing and heating them in a little water until they are soft can help in the extraction of the juice.

Some herbs used for this process are: Aloe vera, chickweed, cilantro, garlic, ginger, *guduchi*, lemon, lime, *neem*, nettles, onion, parsley, *tulsi* (holy basil), turmeric rhizome, *vasa*, and wheatgrass.

Many of these herbs are readily available, but if they are not found fresh, there is another method (although not as potent) for extracting the juice from the dried plant. First the herb is powdered, and then it is soaked in twice its weight of water for 24 hours, after which it can be strained. The dosage of the juice from the fresh plant can be from 1 tsp. to 1 oz., depending upon the potency of the plant used. The fresh juice of a mild tasting plant like *tulsi* can be given in higher quantities than say, ginger root, which is hot and intense.

Herbal Pastes (*Kalka*)

Herbal pastes are prepared by crushing the fresh herb. They are often mixed with various other substances and can be used internally as well as externally as plasters or poultices to promote the healing of sores, boils, rashes, ulcers, and wounds. Any fresh herb may be used in this way. Pastes made from nourishing tonic herbs can also be mixed with nutritive substances like raw sugar, *ghee*, and certain oils to enhance their rejuvenating properties.

Dried powdered herbs can be made into a paste by mixing them with liquids such as water, aloe vera juice, milk, and oils. Herbs can be made more palatable when their powder is mixed with other sweet tasty herbs like licorice or slippery elm, or with substances like raisins, dates, coconut, apricots, and so on. Western herbalists call these preparations electuaries or herbal candies. They are great for the young and old alike. Pastes can also be used as the basis for decoctions and infusions.

Decoctions (*Kvatha*)

This method is best for roots, hard or thick stems, barks, and hard fruits. The process involves boiling 1 part of the herb in 16 parts of water (by weight) over a low flame until only 1/4 remains. If the dry herb is used, then equal parts water can be added to it and left to absorb the water for 1/2 to 1 hour before making the decoction. Then 16 parts water are added before decocting. The whole process can take a fair amount of time depending upon the quantity being prepared. The result is a strong decoction.

In preparing a decoction where different parts of the plant are used, it is best to add roots at the beginning and soft herbs later in the boiling process. Aromatic herbs, tender seeds, and flowers are best added at the end of the boiling process and left to sit in the covered pot, so as not to lose the medicinal properties in the volatile oils of the plant.

To prepare a moderate decoction, the liquid can be reduced to 1/2 of the original amount, and to 3/4 for a weak decoction. Because time is often a factor as to whether a person would take the medicine consistently or not, then reducing the preparation time may be necessary to make it easier. The potency of a decoction will depend on various factors, such as the strength of the person's digestive fire, their state of health, and the severity of the disorder.

Decoctions are usually mixed with jaggary, sugar, honey, medicated *ghee*, or hot water, which act as vehicles to enhance the therapeutic effect of the medicine. Decoctions themselves may be used as vehicles for other medicines as well. The dose for a strong decoction is about 1 oz. It can be doubled or even tripled depending upon the strength of the preparation.

It is best to use earthenware, glass, or suribachi clay pots to make decoctions, although other high quality metal pots are okay, with the exception of aluminum pots, which should never be used for anything except maybe catching water from a leaky roof or changing the oil of a car!

Hot Infusions (*Phanta*)

This method is best for delicate portions of the plant such as stems, soft leaves, small seeds, and flowers. Seeds such as fennel, anise, and cumin can be bruised with a mortar and pestle before adding them to hot water. Infusions are made by pouring about 8 to 16 parts (by volume) of boiling water over 1 to 2 parts of herb (by weight), which are then left to steep in a covered pot for 30 minutes to 8-12 hours. Then the tea is strained and administered. Adding less water will make a stronger infusion.

A convenient method consists in letting the medicine steep all night and using it the next day. A strong infusion is not always necessary. In this case, a 20 to 30 minute infusion can provide wonderful healing benefits, especially when a tea is taken for extended periods of time. This is similar to the standard infusion of Western herbalism. A good method for making a hot infusion is to place a sealed jar of tea in the hot sun for several hours to soak in revitalizing solar energy.

Another preparation of a hot infusion consists in letting the brew sit in hot water for only a short while until it is cool enough to drink. Many Ayurvedic *churnas* (powdered herbs and herbal compounds) are taken in this manner.

Cold Infusion (*Sita Kasaya* or *Hima*)

Cold infusions are made by letting the herb sit in room temperature water, preferably overnight, and then straining well. The same proportions as the hot infusion can be used. Delicate parts of the plant, including leaves, stems, and flowers, are ideal for this process.

Cold infusions are one of the best ways to pacify *pitta*. Herbs like chrysanthemum, coriander, *guduchi*, hibiscus, jasmine, mint, rose petals, and sandalwood work particularly well for this.

Another nice way to make an infusion is to utilize nature's healing energy by letting a tea sit for several hours under the moonlight in an open jar that is sealed with a see-through mesh to imbibe the cooling lunar energy. This is best for calming *pitta*. Both the solar and lunar infusion methods are calming and purifying to the mind. Lunar infusions foster introspection and solar infusion promote transformation and relieve depression.

Additional Plant Preparations

Medicated Wines (*Asavas* and *Arishtas*)

Arishtas are herbal wines made with strong decoctions of various traditional herbal recipes, while *asavas* are made with the juice of the herb or using the herb itself. The herbal concoction is traditionally prepared along with *dhataki* flower (*Woodfordia fruticosa*), which acts as a natural yeast to create fermentation, as well as jaggary and sometimes honey, and then left to sit for 1 month in an earthen vessel or large glass wine jar. A good wine yeast may also be used if *dhataki* is unavailable. Medicinal wines stimulate the digestive fire and are easily digestible. They are often used as vehicles for other medicines. The classical Ayurvedic texts contain many recipes of these wines and their specific indications.

Medicated Milk (*Sidha Dugdham*)

Milk is pacifying to *vata* and *pitta*, and has a calming effect on the body and mind. In Ayurvedic medicine, herbs are often prepared with milk to enhance their nutritive properties or balance their energies. Generally, 1 part of herb is mixed with 8 parts milk and 16 parts water, and boiled down till 1/4 of the liquid remains. Then the decoction is strained and can be mixed with sugar.

For example, 1 oz. of herb is mixed with 1 cup milk and 4 cups water, and boiled till 1 cup remains. This method works especially well to enhance the properties of nourishing and demulcent herbs like *ashwagandha*, *bala*, licorice, *shatavari*, or wild yam. Preparing hot pungent herbs like black pepper, ginger, or *pippali* with milk can help to reduce their hot, sharp qualities and make the milk easier to digest. If powdered herbs are used, then less water may be added in the standard recipe.

A quick method consists in boiling 1 rounded tsp. of the powdered herb in 1 cup of milk and 1/4 cup of water until about 1 cup remains. Many valuable home remedies can be made using this simple method. For instance, a clove of fresh garlic can be decocted using this method, which works well for pacifying *vata* and inducing a sound sleep. Another effective remedy for insomnia or light sleep is *ashwagandha* milk topped with a pinch of nutmeg taken before bedtime. Turmeric or *pippali* milk is helpful for rejuvenating the respiratory tract. *Ashwagandha, bala,* or *shatavari* milk, which are extremely nourishing to the tissues, especially the muscle and reproductive tissues, can be taken in the morning for energy and strength.

Linctus or Jams (*Aveleha, Lehyam, Paka, Prash,* or *Kandha*)

Herbs are also prepared along with jaggary, honey, and *ghee* to make a semi-solid jam. One of the most well known of these confections is the famous *Chyavanprash*, which is an excellent nourishing tonic (*rasayana*) to all the bodily tissues, especially the heart and immune system, and is also used to treat chronic respiratory complaints, general debility, as well as to slow the aging process.

There are a wide variety of jams used in Ayurveda as rejuvenatives. For example, *agastya haritaki* is a jam used to strengthen the lungs and to treat asthma, cough, shortness of breath, hoarseness, consumption, constipation, exhaustion, and piles. *Brahma rasayana* is one of the best jams for rejuvenating the mind and is thought to eliminate fatigue and lethargy, and to promote youthfulness, concentration, intelligence, and longevity.

Pills (*Vati or Gutika*)

There are many Ayurvedic medicines available in pill form in India and abroad, many of which are traditional formulas made from decoctions or dried water extracts, and others are patents created by various Ayurvedic pharmacies. They are often prepared with the resinous herb *guggulu* as well as substances such as sugar or honey, which act as natural binding agents and also contribute their medicinal properties.

One of the unique aspects of many traditional pill preparation is a process known as *bhavana*, where herbs are potentiated by first soaking them in fresh plant juices or strong herbal decoctions. There are different names for pills, depending on their shape and size. The ones shaped like bullets are called *gutika*; tablets are known as *vatika* (or *batika*); and *modaka* refers to balls that are often large in size.

Medicated Oils (*Tailam*)

The method of preparing Ayurvedic medicated oils is quite unique, as it creates highly potent oils, which are not attainable by other simpler infusion techniques. This traditional process consists of decocting 1 part herb (or herbs) with 4 parts oil and 16 parts water over a low heat for several hours (4 to 8 hours, depending on the size of the batch). Toward the end of the process, when the water is almost completely evaporated, it will produce a loud crackling boil, and then subside. At this point, if one drop of water is placed into the remaining oil it will again crackle for a moment, which indicates that the medicated oil is done. Once the oil has cooled down, it is strained through a fine mesh, muslin bag, or straining sock (available at wine making supply stores).

Another way to prepare the oil is to first decoct the herb in the water until 1/4 of the water remains, and strain the remaining liquid well. At this point, an equal quantity of oil is added and the process completed as mentioned above. This method helps to prevent any herbs from burning at the bottom of the pot and also makes it easier to hear when the last bit of moisture is about to evaporate.

A simple oil infusion can be made by placing 1 part herb into 4 parts oil left to sit in a sealed jar for up to 1 month. If fresh herbs are used, then it is helpful to mince before placing them in the oil. This is a fine method for making mild strength oils, particularly when using highly aromatic herbs or fresh leaves and flowers, although dry herbs can also be used.

A similar result to that of the simple oil infusion can be achieved by a solar oil infusion, which is done by placing the jar containing the herbs and oil outside in the sunlight for 4 to 5 hours a day, during the warmest times of the day, for 3 to 4 weeks. Some of the best herbs used for simple infusions include arnica, calendula, garlic, mullein, and St. John's wort.

A hot oil infusion can be made by mixing 1 part herb with 4 parts oil, bringing it to a boil, immediately removing it from the heat, then covering the pot and letting it steep for 12 hours. After straining well, it can be stored in an airtight glass jar.

Sesame oil is the most common base oil used in the preparation of *tailams*, although other oils, such as coconut, almond, sunflower, and castor oil are also used in certain preparations. *Tailams* are also used for nasal application (*nasya*), oil enema (*anuvasan basti*), douche (*ut-*

tara basti), ointment for the eyes and ears, and some may also be taken orally.

Medicated oils play a central role in Ayurveda. Massaging oils into the body facilitates balancing the *doshas* and removing toxins. It also helps to kindle the *dhatu agni*, the digestive fire of each of the tissues, to calm the mind, relax the body, and refresh the spirit.

Common daily Ayurvedic practices consist in applying a small amount of warm oil to the scalp and soles before going to bed, as well as a daily self-massage with oil before a warm morning shower. (See *Dinacharya*.)

Medicated *Ghee* (*Siddha Ghritam*)

Ghee, or clarified butter, can be bought in most health food and Indian grocery stores, or easily made at home to assure quality and purity, especially when used for medicinal purposes. To prepare plain *ghee*, melt 1 lb. of unsalted—preferably organic—butter in a medium saucepan, bring to a light boil over a low flame, and allow it to cook for 15 minutes or so. Foam will rise to the top, but should not be removed during the cooking process, because it contains medicinal properties. The solids will settle to the bottom of the pan and will eventually turn to a light tan color. The *ghee* will give off popcorn like fragrance, indicating that it is ready. At this point, turn off the heat and once it has cooled a bit strain the *ghee* through a super fine strainer or a few layers of cheesecloth and store in an airtight jar. If *ghee* is prepared properly, with all the moisture and lactose cooked out, it does not require refrigeration.

Ghee alleviates *vata* and *pitta doshas*. It kindles the digestive fire without aggravating *pitta*, strengthens immunity by enhancing and protecting *ojas* (the refined essence of the bodily tissues), and nourishes the mind and nervous system. *Ghee* also acts a *yogavahi*, or catalytic agent that helps to carry the medicinal properties of herbs to the seven *dhatus*. There is a variety of medicinal *ghees* or *ghritams* used in Ayurvedic medicine, and many Western herbs can be used in making such medicines as well. The process for preparing medicated *ghee* is the same decoction method used to make medicated oils.

Herbal Powder (*Churna*)

Ayurveda uses many herbs in powdered form because they are quick to infuse and easy to administer. A typical dose is 1/2 to 1 tsp., which can be infused into hot or cool water. Powders are convenient and useful in clinical practice for making formulas on the spot to meet the specific needs of an individual. A wide variety of traditional Ayurvedic compounds are made of powdered herbs, and some of them can also be purchased in tablet or capsule form.

One drawback to powdered herbs is that they tend to lose their potency quicker (6 to 12 months) than whole or cut herbs, so it is good not to store more than you think you will need for a year's time. However, when certain herbal formulas are prepared with Ayurvedic alchemical substances (see *bhasmas* below), they can last a very long time. If herbs are made into tablets, they retain their potency for at least double the time of that of loose powders. *Guggulu* compounds keep their potency for several years when stored in a dark, cool, and dry environment.

Alchemical Mineral and Metal Preparations (*Bhasmas* and *Rasa Rasayanas*)

Ayurveda possesses one of the oldest forms of alchemy, known as *rasa shastra*. Many minerals and metals are used as medicine after being subjected to highly specialized processes to draw out their toxic elements, including that of incineration and soaking in various substances. These preparations are called *bhasmas*, which are super fine ashes with subtle yet extremely powerful healing properties.

Preparations known as *rasa rasayanas* are made by humanizing substances such as sulfur and mercury into very powerful yet safe and effective medicines. These alchemical substances are often mixed with herbs, as they have the power to enhance the action a thousand times and carry the properties of the herbs they are mixed with deep into the tissues of the body. They also help to preserve herbal formulas for as long as a lifetime. These alchemical medicines are still widely used in India but have been restricted in the Western world.

Guggulu Compounds

These are a class of special medicines that contain *guggulu* (*Commiphora mukul*), which is a purifying and rejuvenating tree resin. They are available in both powder and pill form and are used to treat a wide variety of *vata* and *kapha* complaints relating to the joints and nervous system.

Guggulu is added to many formulas as a binding agent of pills and tablets. It is also a *yogavahi*, or catalytic agent that enhances the action of herbs it is combined with and carries their properties to the deep tissue layers. There are many *guggulu* compounds used in

Ayurvedic medicine to treat various disorders, such as arthritic conditions, accumulations of excess *kapha* and *ama*, and diseases of the nervous system. (See *Traditional Herbal Compounds*.)

Utensils Used for Preparation

When preparing herbs, it is important to have the proper utensils at your disposal, such as cooking pots, measuring cups and spoons, a scale (ounce and gram), a fine strainer, cheese cloth, and a straining sock.

Since ancient times, earthen cookware has been the cooking vessel of choice. Ceramic, glass, and suribachi clay pots are ideal, although in Ayurveda high quality metallic pots, such as stainless steel or enamel, may also be used. Never use aluminum or non-stick pots because they are toxic to the body.

Certain metallic drinking vessels are used to increase the effects of water or herbal teas upon a specific *dosha*. For instance, drinking from a copper cup reduces *kapha,* because copper has *lechana*, or scraping action. A silver cup is best for decreasing *pitta*, since silver is cooling. A clay or pottery cup can be grounding for *vata*. Stainless steel cups are *tridoshic* in action.

The Art of Formulation

When it comes to herbal formulation, there is strength in numbers. The power of a single herb can be greatly potentiated when combined with other herbs that share similar actions. Herbal compounding is not unique to Ayurveda, but Ayurveda's theoretical framework provides a valuable tool for choosing herbs appropriately, from a constitutional perspective. There are a number of principles to consider when creating any herbal compound.

The principle of synergy arises from the idea that combining herbs with similar actions enhances their therapeutic effects. There is usually a main herb, and herbs possessing similar properties are added to support it. A single herb often has many different properties, so the overall action of a compound depends primarily upon the similarity of the herbs used in it. For instance, if the formula is going to be directed at the liver and blood, then herbs such as burdock or *guduchi* may be chosen as the main herb, and herbs like milk thistle or *neem* could be used as supports.

Next, assisting herbs can be added to target secondary symptoms and complaints. For example, if there is an inflammatory skin condition like psoriasis, then herbs that help to calm itching, like turmeric or *manjista*, which also have an affinity to the liver and blood, can be added to the formula.

Furthermore, stimulant and carminative herbs can be mixed in to act as carrying herbs to enhance the digestion, absorption, and assimilation of the compound. Carrying herbs are typically heating and used in smaller amounts than the main herbs. The Ayurvedic compound *trikatu*, which contains black pepper, ginger, and *pippali*, is often used for this purpose. Such herbs are especially important when a compound contains several nutritive tonic herbs, which often have sweet, heavy, and cooling qualities that can decrease the power of *agni* and promote the accumulation of *ama* if they are not digested properly.

Another important principle to consider in compounding is that of opposition. When the qualities of a particular formula are too strong, other herbs can be added to create a counter balancing or antagonizing effect. For example, when a compound contains several bitter herbs, it can cause cold and dry qualities to accumulate, which may eventually weaken the digestive fire and deplete bodily tissues. Here warming herbs like ginger or cinnamon can minimize these cold qualities, and demulcent herbs like licorice or marshmallow, which are moistening, can prevent dryness.

Adding a small amount of eliminatory herbs helps to prevent the build up of toxins, caused either by certain herbs or from toxins moving out of the body as a result of cleansing herbal treatments. For such purposes, diuretic and laxative herbs are used to cleanse wastes via the large intestine and urinary tract. With this in mind, the Ayurvedic compound *triphala* is commonly used in many formulas, whereas in Western herbalism, herbs like cascara sagrada or rhubarb are often used.

Principles of Constitutional Formulation

Creating constitutional formulas follows much of the same principles as making compounds. The basic strategy is to choose several herbs with properties that address key aspects of the individual case, such as the main *doshic* imbalance, symptoms, quality of digestion and elimination, as well as the tissues, organs, and channels involved. Constitutional formulas create an energetic signature that resonates with the totality of the individual and help strengthen the communication between cells, tissues, and organs throughout the entire organism. In this sense, the herbs are not meant to heal in and of themselves, but rather to restore and stimulate the body's own ability to heal itself.

Because a single herb can have many properties, herbs can be chosen to address more than one particular element of the overall treatment. This can help keep the total number of herbs in a formula to a minimum, and it also keeps the focus of the formula from becoming too general. With this in mind, it is important to follow a few fundamental principles of constitutional formulation, which are rooted in basic Ayurvedic theory.

First, the main herb or herbs selected for a formula should be *dosha pratyanika*, which means specific to the predominant *dosha* of the constitution, or the causative *dosha* in the disease process. Next come herbs that are *vyadhi pratyanika*, i.e., specific to the nature of the disease or disorder. Other herbs can be added to address *lakshanami*, or specific signs and symptoms, whether physical, mental, or emotional. Furthermore, herbs can be selected to balance and maintain the normal function of *agni,* digestion and elimination, as well as the health of the organs and channels involved.

A well-balanced formula can serve as a good foundation and help to reduce the number of traditional or patent compounds needed for treatment. Depending on the severity of the case, a more direct action may be needed. Here specific compounds can be used along with the constitutional formula.

If using only separate compounds or patent formulas, the same principles can be followed. Ultimately, the key is to choose the least amount of compounds to cover the most ground possible. Bombarding the organism with too many patent formulas may prove counter productive, as the person may not be able to digest so much medicine at once. This is why constitutional formulas can be extremely valuable, and herbal formulation an art to be mastered.

The healing properties of herbs come from more than their chemical constituents. In fact, the ancient *rishis* and sages of India, who were Ayurvedic masters, didn't view nature through the lens of biochemistry. They gained knowledge of plants though direct perception and experience. They observed how a plant looked, where it grew, how it tasted, what its energies, post-digestive effects, and even special and spiritual potencies were. The taste of a substance alone has the power to immediately shift the content of our consciousness through its sublingual action. So, with this in mind, we must remember that a simple formula that resonates with the needs of the whole person (i.e. body, mind, and spirit) can produce remarkable results, and that often times less can be more.

Important Tips for Formulation

Proportions

To ensure the desired effects of a formula, it is important to choose the appropriate proportions for each of the herbs used. Typically, the main and supporting herbs will make up the bulk of the formula. Next, in terms of quantity, come the assisting herbs. The amount of herb used to counter balance a formula will vary, depending upon the qualities of the herbs used, but it will be less than the main and supporting herbs and sometimes less than the assisting herbs as well. Last but not least, come the carrying and eliminating herbs, which are usually added in small amounts. There are no hard and fast rules when it comes to proportions, and each herbalist has his or her own approach.

Treating the Whole Person

The body expresses and points to what is happening at a deeper level through signs and symptoms. If we focus on the finger that points to the moon, we will only see the finger and miss the moon. Likewise, if we only address symptoms and disregard the underlying cause, then we will miss the bigger picture and will not be able to get to the root of the problem and cure. Furthermore, if we try to treat every single symptom, then the properties of the herbs can easily become too diverse and their actions too diluted to yield the desired result. In Ayurveda, symptoms are viewed as qualitative expressions of a *doshic* imbalance, so if balance is restored at a *doshic* level, symptoms will disappear on their own. Removing the root of a tree will take care of the branches as well.

Reduction or Tonic Therapy

Before choosing or creating a formula, it is important to consider the strength of the individual and whether or not *ama* is present. If there is generalized weakness, then nutritive and rejuvenating tonic herbs may be needed. If *ama* is present, then reduction therapy will be indicated to promote cleansing. In some situations, there may be a need to do reduction as well as tonification. In this case, a formula can have elements of both actions with an emphasis on the action that is most needed. For instance, if there is a need to burn and eliminate toxins, but the person is also deficient in certain areas, then some tonic herbs may be added as supporting or assisting herbs to prevent weakening the individual even further.

Keeping It Simple

Herbs have a broad spectrum of action. Adding too many without a clear objective can weaken the effects of a compound. Similarly, when designing an herbal regime, it is best not to recommend too many different formulas. This approach becomes too diluted and sends mixed messages to the body.

There are some Ayurvedic compounds that contain a large number of herbs, but the key to their effectiveness lies in the skill with which they have been formulated. Again, there is no hard and fast rule on how to formulate, but in my experience some of the most remarkable results come from simple constitutional formulas and a select few of the most appropriate compounds.

Energizing Herbs with Mantra

Mantras contain sacred *bija* (seed) syllables that help to purify the mind and subtle body, and have remarkable healing powers. The ancient *rishis* and yogis perceived that each part of the body resonates with a specific sound or *bija* mantra. Furthermore, each of the sounds that make up the Sanskrit alphabet resonates with every part of the body. Likewise, herbs have subtle vibrations. This is why Ayurvedic herbs are often harvested and prepared while specific mantras are recited. Chanting mantras when mixing or preparing herbs helps to infuse the herbs with more *prana* (vital energy) and with the healing intention of the person chanting.

The mantra to the Divine Mother, also known as *Navarna Mantra*, can be used to bring divine energy into foods and medicinal substances. It is a prayer to the various aspects of the Divine Mother (Saraswati, Laxmi, Kali, and Durga). It can be repeated while preparing herbs or food.

"Om Aim Hreem Kleem Chamundaya Vichchay"

Repetition of mantra can also go beyond the physical recitation of sacred syllables. Yogis have taught that the movement of the breath makes the mantra *So Ham*, which can be translated as *I Am*, and is the first expression of primordial matter, or *Prakruti*, as the Cosmic Intellect. Each inhalation creates the subtle sound *So* and each exhalation the sound *Ham* (pronounced *Hum*). Our awareness of the breath is the thread that links each and every moment like beads in a strand. If we can maintain this awareness in our daily life, it will greatly increase our healing power at the physical, mental, and spiritual levels. Ayurvedic practitioners can also consciously use this

So Ham mantra to enhance their awareness during pulse diagnosis. Simply pay attention to the sound *So* while inhaling and the sound *Ham* (*Hum*) while exhaling.

The Aim of Treatment

In Ayurveda, the maintenance of health and the treatment of disease are always seen in relation to the three *doshas*, which make up the individual constitution. It is at the constitutional level that true healing takes place and not by simply focusing on the signs and symptoms of disease. No two beings are exactly alike, and the causes leading to imbalance, both physically and psychologically, are unique. Therefore, the path toward optimal health has to be individualized.

Ayurveda views that symptoms are the body's way of expressing a *doshic* imbalance, so they tell the practitioner what is happening at a deeper level. Obviously, if we treat two people with the same chronic disorder both treatments may share some similarities, but each approach will be different and unique, depending on individual factors. In other words, we have to aim at restoring balance at a constitutional level in order to address the root cause of a chronic disease.

Routes of Administration of Herbs

Typically, herbs are administered in tea or pill form, but depending upon the nature and location of the disorder, there are specific routes of administration that can provide a more direct effect upon a particular region of the body and *doshic* condition. Listed below are the main routes of administration used in Ayurveda.

Basti (Enema Therapy)

There are three main types of *basti*: Herbal decoction (*niruha*), oil enema (*anuvasana*), and vaginal douche (*uttara basti*). *Basti* therapy acts directly on the colon, which is the main site of *vata dosha*, and also where any medicinal substances are absorbed and carried throughout the entire body. This therapy removes excess *vata* and *ama* from the colon and encourages the *vata* that has spread into the deeper tissues, such as the musculoskeletal or nervous system, to return to its main site to be eliminated. It can also be used to treat other *doshic* imbalances, especially those affecting the pelvic region. In fact, since *vata* is often involved in many disorders, either as the primary or secondary *dosha*, *basti* therapy plays a primary role in the treatment of almost all disease, especially during a *Panchakarma* program.

Ayurvedic enemas are not the same as a high enema or colonic therapy, which use large amounts of liquid, often to evacuate the entire colon. These therapies tend to create more space for *vata* to expand and become aggravated, and if done too frequently, they wash away healthy intestinal flora.

Conversely, *basti* is generally given in small amounts (from 1 to 2 cups of liquid) at a time. It is gentle and can be administered on a daily basis during cleansing programs without depleting the body, and sometimes weekly in the management of certain conditions. The herbs and substances used, as well as the frequency and duration of the therapy, depend upon the *doshic* involvement and specific disorder, and also the strength and constitution of the person.

Sesame oil and sweet, nourishing, and tonifying herbs are often used to help treat a wide variety of *vata* conditions. Although enemas are primarily used for pacifying excess *vata*, they can be beneficial for *pitta* and *kapha* disorders as well. Sweet, bitter, and astringent herbs and substances like milk or buttermilk help to treat *pitta* related conditions like ulcerative colitis and Crohn's disease. Pungent herbs reduce *kapha* and help to remove *ama*, mucus, and food masses from the colon. Pure oil enemas are used to treat dry conditions, nervous disorders, and degenerative types of *vata* diseases. Decoctions help to remove *dosha* and *ama* from the *srotamsi*, or bodily channels. Small amounts of oil are often added to decoctions for a more dynamic action. During a longer series of treatments, alternating between plain oil enemas and decoction enemas is preferred, always ending on the last day with oil.

Douching is another form of *basti*, and is used for disorders of the urinary tract, bladder, vagina, and uterus. This method doesn't disturb the beneficial bacteria of the vagina when used appropriately and not in excess. Depending on the given situation, mild infusions of herbs such as licorice, rose petals, raspberry leaf, and *shatavari*, as well as medicines such as *tikta ghritam*, are used with this method.

Nasya (Nasal Administration)

Nasal administration of herbs includes medicated oils and *ghee*, *neti* (salt water nasal flushing), inhalation of herbal vapors or powders, and aromatherapy with essential oils. *Nasya* therapy is used to restore the balance and function of *prana vayu*, which governs the mind, senses, and nervous system, as well as respiratory functions. It helps to remove excess *dosha* and *ama* that has accumulated in the head, sinuses, nose, and throat. Certain *nasya* therapies also help to release suppressed emotions and relieve pain and tension along the spine.

Nasyas containing pungent herbs like ginger and eucalyptus help to purge phlegm. Those with nervines like gotu kola, calamus, and skullcap have a direct action on the brain and nervous system, especially when prepared in a medicated *ghee*. *Ghee* or sesame oil can also be administered alone, and are useful for treating dry nasal passageways. Simply applying *ghee* to the nostrils creates a protective coating, which can alleviate allergies to dusts, molds, and pollen. A typical dose for *nasya* oils or medicated *ghee* is 1 to 5 drops in each nostril (although more can be used for specific conditions) while laying flat on the back with the head slightly tilted back. Another method known as *pratimarsha* consists in applying the *nasya* oil to the pinky finger and gently inserting it into each nostril while massaging it in a twisting motion. This can help to prevent or correct mild deviation of the septum and free up blocked emotions.

Dhuman (Smoking of Herbs)

In Ayurveda, smoking of herbs is used to decongest the lungs and relieve cough. Herbs like calamus (*vacha*), gotu kola, *jyotishmati*, and passion flower can be smoked to calm and rejuvenate the mind. Other herbs like coltsfoot, mullein, peppermint, and turmeric are smoked to relieve congestion and cough. Herbs like *shardunika* or lobelia, when added to cigarettes can help to diminish the craving for smoking. Likewise, a pinch of calamus can be added to marijuana to help minimize its *vata* provoking effects. Herbs should not be smoked too often due to the tar and particles that result from burning the plant.

In the Native American tradition, tobacco smoke is believed to carry or clear subtle energies, and is used to purify the atmosphere and the mind, as well as to carry prayers to the Great Spirit.

Typical herbs used for smoking are: *Ajwan*, bayberry, black pepper, calamus, cardamom, catnip, cinnamon, cloves, cubebs, ginger, gotu kola, hops, lemonbalm, lobelia, mint (all), mugwort, passion flower, sage, and turmeric.

Karana Purana (Filling the Ears)

This therapy involves administering either plain or medicated oil into the ears. This is done, depending on the case, by applying just a few drops or filling the whole ear. This method is used to treat diseases of the ear, earaches, deafness, ringing in the ears, headaches, insomnia, neck and shoulder stiffness, wry neck, lock jaw, misalignment of the spine, and giddiness. A simple method of pacifying *vata* in the ears is to fill each ear with lukewarm sesame oil while lying on the side and retaining the oil for 10 to 20 minutes. If this therapy is performed on another person, it is beneficial to massage the *marmas* (energy points) on and around the ear while the ear is full of oil. The right ear should always be treated first.

Another method of *karana purana* consists in placing a small amount of warm oil into the ear before bedtime and allowing it to be absorbed throughout the night, alternating ears each night. Caution should be used if there is an ear infection, when only a few drops of medicated oil, such as tea tree (essential oil), garlic, mullein, or *bilva,* are indicated.

Ashcotana-Anjana (Eye Administration)

Herbal medicines can be used for disorders of the eyes and applied to the eyes in the form of drops, ointments, *ghee*, herbal eyewashes, and oils. One method of nourishing and rejuvenating the eyes is *netra basti*, which consists in bathing the eyes in *ghee*. Here a dam is formed around the eye with a dough made from grain flour such as wheat, and then filled with slightly warmed *ghee*. The person then opens the eye, allowing the eyeball to completely bathe in the *ghee*. This therapy helps to calm aggravated *doshas* in the head, improve the eyesight, relieve eyestrain, and is very effective in treating various diseases of the eyes. Another simple way of cleansing and nourishing the eyes is to apply 1 drop of pure castor oil or *ghee* into each eye at bedtime. Castor oil helps to prevent cataracts and treat it in its early stages, and *ghee* is cooling and relieves eye strain. Other herbs used for eye drops include chamomile, *punarnava*, rose water, and *triphala churna*.

Topical Applications

Ayurveda has a wide variety of topical applications of herbs and oils. The skin is the largest organ of the body and a major gateway for receiving the medicinal properties of all substances, so many herbs and oils are used on the skin in the form of pastes, poultices, boluses, and medicated and scented oils. When herbs are used in this manner, they also help to pull impurities out of the body.

Herbal plastering, or *lepa*, is often used to calm skin rashes, draw out infections, and promote the healing of wounds and sores. Sometimes pastes are applied over the entire body, as during *Panchakarma,* to tone the skin and pull out toxins and excess *dosha*. Cooling herbs have *pitta* pacifying effects and help to reduce inflammation and calm itching. Nervine herbs can be applied to the soles to calm *vata* conditions of the nervous system. Bitter and astringent herbs can help to relieve swelling due to excess *kapha*.

For daily washing of the skin, Ayurveda recommends *ubtans* (herbal scrubs), which are mixtures of herb, bean flours, and oils that can be used with warm water instead of soap. *Ubtans* can be made with ingredients such as lentil flour, chickpea flour, barley flour, sandalwood powder, rose petals, turmeric powder, saffron, almond oil, lemon oil, and so on. They can also be specifically formulated for *vata, kapha*, or *pitta* type of skin, or to address specific needs and skin conditions.

One of the most important topical therapies in Ayurveda is massaging medicated oils into the body. An effective topical application to pacify *vata* consists in massaging with sesame oil, which can be done daily as a self-massage before a warm shower.

There are other topical therapies similar to *netra basti*, where oils are pooled onto specific areas of the body. The main ones are: *Shiro basti* for the top of the head, *hrud* (or *uro*) *basti* for the heart, and *kati basti* for the lumbo-sacral area.

Anupanas or Media of Intake

In Ayurvedic medicine, herbs are often administered along with various *anupanas*, or media of intake, such as hot or cool water, honey, *ghee*, fruit juices, broths, teas, sugar, or warm milk. *Anupanas* help to enhance and support the effect of the herbs they are given with. They have an affinity to specific tissues, so they can act as a *yogavahi* (catalytic agents) to guide the action of herbs more directly. Because herbs can possess a wide range of properties, *anupanas* can direct them to have a more specific action. For example, cow's or goat's milk is used to target *vata* in the bone tissue in cases of osteoporosis, and a bitter herb like burdock can be given along with aloe vera gel to enhance its alterative properties.

Anupanas may also help to influence which *dosha* an herb or formula will have the most effect on. As a general rule, hot water or heating substances are going to pacify *vata* and *kapha*, whereas cool water or substances will pacify *pitta*. Typical *anupanas* for pacifying *vata* are sesame oil, *ghee*, butter, ginger tea, and hot milk or water. *Ghee*, aloe vera, milk, pomegranate juice, coriander tea, and cool water are *pitta* pacifying. Good stimulating *anupanas* to reduce *kapha* are hot water, honey, *guggulu*, and dried ginger tea.

Anupanas can also be used to target specific *dhatus* (tissues). It is hard to limit a substance to one specific *dhatu*, but below are a few examples of the common usâge of *anupanas*.

Milk is used to target *rasa dhatu* (plasma and lymph) and *rakta dhatu* (blood); milk also has an affinity to the bone and reproductive tissues. Milk is sweet, cooling, calming, and nourishing. Therefore, it is used to enhance rejuvenating herbs and to prevent heating herbs from aggravating *pitta*. Milk used with nervine sedative herbs helps to induce a sound sleep.

Water is also used to target the plasma and blood tissues. Hot water is a good *anupana* for diaphoretic herbs to induce sweating and for digestive stimulating herbs to kindle *agni* and burn *ama*. Cool water helps to bring out the diuretic properties of herbs as well as the *pitta* pacifying effects of bitter herbs.

Honey acts on the blood, muscle, and fat tissues. Honey has a scraping action *(lekaniya)* and when given along with stimulating or expectorant herbs, it brings out their *kapha* reducing properties.

Aloe vera nourishes all *dhatus*, but has a special affinity to the plasma, blood, and reproductive tissues. Aloe vera juice or gel is one of the most common *anupanas* used along with *pitta* pacifying herbs and formulas.

Alcohol (as used in medicated wines, extracts, and tinctures) quickly affects the nerve tissue due to its light, subtle, and penetrating qualities.

G*hee* has a special affinity to the fat tissue, but can act on all *dhatus*.

Herbal decoctions and infusions can also be used as *anupanas*. For instance, a tea made with the compound *trikatu*, which is composed of black pepper, ginger, and *pippali*, can be used to enhance other *kapha* pacifying medicines. Likewise, peppermint, chamomile, or ginger tea can assist herbs used for digestive complaints.

***Anupanas* for *vata*:** Hot water or milk, plain and medicated *ghee*, sesame oil, raw sugar, chamomile.

***Anupanas* for *pitta*:** Aloe vera, pomegranate juice, bitter teas, plain or bitter *ghee*, cool water, milk, peppermint, *sita* (rock candy), cooling bitter herbal teas.

***Anupanas* for *kapha*:** Honey, hot water, hot pungent herbal teas.

Timing of Administration of Herbs

In Ayurvedic herbology, the timing of administration of a medicine is another important factor to consider, as it may enhance its effects. Herbs that are taken before meals work more on the colon, kidneys, and reproductive organs, and play a key role in supporting the functions of *apana vayu*, the downward moving aspect of *vata* that governs elimination of waste products and menstruation. Herbs with mild laxative, diuretic, and emmenagogue properties also act on the lower half of the body, and can be taken before food to strengthen their action.

Herbs taken along with food act directly upon the stomach, spleen, liver, and small intestine. They support *samana vayu*, the aspect of *vata* governing digestive functions, as well as *jathara agni* and *pachaka pitta*, the main fires of digestion in the stomach and small intestine. Herbs acting on the middle part of the body are carminatives, stimulants, bitters, and nutritive tonics. Herbs taken after meals work on the upper portion of the body and directly affect *prana, udana,* and *vyana vayus*, giving them a stronger action on the lungs, heart, brain, and nervous system.Below is a list of times of administration and the therapeutic effect they enhance.

Anannakala: Empty Stomach

Herbs taken first thing in the morning, then allowing as much time as possible (1-3 hours) before taking food, help to increase *agni* and burn *ama* and phlegm. This is a good time to enhance various properties such as *lekaniya* (scraping of fat). This is the ideal time to give purgatives, emetics, or *rasayanas* (rejuvenating substances).

Pragbhukta: Before Meals

Herbs taken at this time are carried quickly to the pelvic region and have the greatest effect on the colon and *apana vayu*. This is one of the best times for treating chronic indigestion, gas, bloating, abdominal discomfort, and constipation, as well as disorders of the reproductive organs and urinary tract.

Madhyabhukta: During Meals

Herbs taken along with food act on *samana vayu*, the aspects of *vata* governing digestive functions in the area of the duodenum and small intestine. This is helpful for kindling the *agni*, improving peristalsis, absorption, and assimilation. It is also an easier way of taking herbs for those who have difficulty swallowing them or tolerating their taste.

Adhobhukta: Right After Meals

Herbs taken just after food work on the upper portion of the body and directly affect *prana vayu*, the aspect of *vata* governing respiration and the nervous system. They also help to restore the function of *udana*, the *vayu* responsible for speech, effort, energy, willpower, and memory, as well as that of *vyana vayu*, which is centered in the heart, moves throughout the body, and governs circulation. Digestive herbs can also be taken at this time to treat slow sluggish digestion and help to strengthen and regulate the thyroid gland. People that are sensitive to herbs sometimes prefer to take herbs after meals. This seems to be a convenient time for people to remember to take their herbs, but proper timing should be encouraged whenever possible.

Antarabhukta: Between Meals

The seven bodily tissues receive their nourishment during this time (3 to 4 hours after a meal). Herbs taken at this time travel along with *ahara rasa* (nutrient precursors) to each of the *dhatus*, increasing metabolic activity.

Muhur Muhur: Frequent Administration

This can be as frequent as moment to moment or every few minutes. This method helps to send a constant reminder to the body. It is used for acute disorders of *prana vayu* like hiccup, burping, asthma, cough, and other respiratory disorders. Good examples of this are sipping on teas every 5-10 minutes, or licking certain pastes made from herbs and substances like honey to relieve acute symptoms. Another example is the use of spice blends for digestion (digestive *churnas*), which can be sprinkled on food and ingested every few minutes with each bite.

Swapnakala: Before Bedtime

Herbs given at bedtime or one hour before sleep help to redirect the movement of *vata* (*vata anuloman*). This is a good time to give laxatives or purgatives, and is also an ideal time for treating insomnia and other sleep disorders. Herbs taken at midnight can help with nightmares and disorders of *majja dhatu* (nerve tissue and marrow).

Sandhyakale: At Sunrise and Sunset

Herbs taken during this time act directly on the joints. Mild laxatives can also be taken at sunrise. Herbs that raise the consciousness, such as *brahmi* and *vacha*, can be taken in the early morning to promote good meditation.

Patient Compliance

Some people find it difficult to take herbs at different times due to their lifestyles, especially when they need to take several medicines at different times of the day. For this reason, many practitioners recommend taking the main medicines at whatever time is most convenient. This is not the ideal method of administration, but it is better to take the medicine than to skip doses, or worse, to give up on an herbal program that seems too difficult to integrate into one's lifestyle.

Dosage and Preparation

In Ayurveda, the method of herbal preparation and dosage is individualized to meet the overall needs of the person. Factors such as the age, constitution, strength of digestion, level of *ama*, body weight, and severity of the disorder should be taken into consideration when designing a treatment plan. Other considerations play an important role as well, such as understanding which *doshas* are involved, their qualitative expressions, level of involvement and direction, as well as which tissues, channels, and organs they are affecting.

Taste can also be an indicator of the proper dosage of an herb. Sweet herbs are heavy and nourishing to the bodily tissues, so they can often be given in moderate to large dosages, providing that the *agni* is strong enough to digest them. Hot and pungent herbs like black pepper or cayenne should be given in lower dosages, due to their hot, sharp, and intense actions. Bitter herbs, for the most part, are cooling and can be depleting to the digestive fire and the bodily tissues when used in excess. Therefore, they should be used in small to moderate dosages and well balanced with other herbs when given for long periods. (See also *The Art of Formulation*.)

If the digestive fire is low, or if *ama* is present in the GI track, then strong dosages of herbs may not be digested properly, which will cause more *ama* to form as a result, and can further aggravate the condition. In such cases, it is good to start with a mild dosage and also to give herbs that will stimulate *agni* and burn *ama*, such as hot pungent herbs. For young children and the elderly, mild dosages are always indicated. Listed below are some common methods of preparation for the intake of herbs and herbal formulas, with recommended dosage.

Decoction

The decoction method is used to extract the constituents from the hard portions of the plant (roots, bark, hard stems and leaves, and seeds). When making decoctions, the pot should be uncovered while the herbs are simmering. This method is more time consuming, but produces a strong acting brew. If a selected formula contains both hard and soft portions of plants, then the softer portions (tender leaves, stems, and flowers) can be added at the end of the simmering process and left to steep for at least 1/2 hour.

Strong decoction: Use 4 oz. of herb per 1/2 gallon of water and boil over a low flame until the liquid is reduced to 1 pint (16 fl oz.).

Dosage: 1/4 cup, 2-3 times a day.

Medium decoction: Use 2 to 4 oz. of herb per 1 quart of water and boil with the lid on, over a low flame, until 1 pint remains (16 fl oz.).

Dosage: 1/2 to 1 cup, 2-3 times a day.

Mild decoction: Add 1 to 2 oz. of herb to 1 quart of water and lightly boil with the lid on, over a low flame, for 20 to 30 minutes. This method, commonly used in Western herbalism, is simple and effective.

Dosage: 1/2 to 1 cup, 2-4 times a day.

Infusions

Strong infusion: Pour 1 quart of boiling water over 4 oz. of herb, cover tightly, and allow it to steep for an hour or more, if desired. This method works best for cut and sifted herbs.

Dosage: 1/4 to 1/2 cup, 3 times a day.

Medium infusion: This is the same method as the strong infusion, but using only 2 oz. of herb to 1 quart of boiling water.

Dosage: 1/4 to 1/2 cup, 2-3 times a day.

Mild infusion: Use 1/2 to 1 oz. of herb per quart (or 1 heaping tablespoon to 1 cup) of boiling water.

Dosage: 1 cup, 3 times daily.

Cold infusion (*sita phant*)**:** This method is similar to the previous ones, except that room temperature water is used instead of boiling water, and it can be left to steep overnight. It can be made in mild, medium, or strong potencies.

Preparations for Daily Use

When herbs need to be taken on a daily basis and over a long period, a simple method using powdered or finely cut herbs can be chosen. This preparation may not provide the same potency as a stronger infusion, but it is simple and easy for most people, since it can be done pretty much anywhere.

Simple Infusion

Medium to strong infusion: Mix 3 to 6 gm (1 to 2 tsp.) of herb into 1 cup hot water and let it set till it is drinking temperature. If powdered herbs are used, stir well and drink powder and all. If cut herbs are used, strain before drinking.

Dosage: 1 cup, 2 to 3 times a day.

Mild infusion: Infuse 1/4 to 1/2 tsp. of herb per 1 cup of hot water.

Dosage: 1 cup, 2 to 3 times a day.

Simple Decoction

Add 1 to 2 tsp. (3 to 6 gm) of herb to 1-1/2 cup of water and boil in a covered pot until 1 cup of liquid remains.

Dosage: 2 to 3 times daily.

Pills and Capsules

Ayurveda recommends that herbs be tasted, because the first action of an herb is through its taste on the tongue. So, if possible, it is best to chew pills and tablets a little to taste the herbs and aid in their digestion. However, taking capsules or pills may be the only way for some people to take herbs, which is still better than not taking them at all. One "OO" sized capsule holds approximately 250 mg of powdered herb, so 2 to 4 capsules provide a sufficient adult dosage and can be given 2 to 3 times daily. For children 1 to 2 capsules, 2 to 3 times daily, is sufficient. If "OO" capsules are too big for small children to swallow, then "O" capsules can be used.

Simple Conversion Method

The weight of a ground herb will vary depending upon its density, as well as how finely ground it is. When formulating with powdered herbs, it is easier and quicker to measure in parts rather than by weight. This can be done with a measuring teaspoon, a tablespoon, or any measuring utensil, depending upon the quantity being prepared.

For instance, dense, resinous, or finely ground herbs can be measured at a shy to a leveled teaspoon, whereas with herbs with more of a light or fluffy consistency, the measure can be slightly rounded. For clinical practice, I prefer using an ounce/gram scale to insure total accuracy of each herb or substance in a formula with a simple conversion method like the one listed below.

60 drops of liquid = 1 tsp.

1 tsp. (powdered herb) = 2.5 to 3 g

2 tsp. (powdered herb) = 5 to 6 g

3 tsp. (powdered herb) = 7 to 9 g

Medicinal Herbs (East and West)

[Materia Medica]

AJWAN

Trachyapermum copticum; Umbelliferae

AJMODA

Apium graveolens; Umbelliferae

CAROM, WILD CELERY

Effect on Doshas: V- P+ K-
Rasa: pungent, bitter **Virya:** heating **Vipak:** pungent
Preparations: infusion (powder), decoction (seed), oil.
Dosage: 1-3 g per day.

Parts used: seeds, roots.

Tissues: plasma, blood, fat, nerve and marrow, reproductive.

Systems: digestive, nervous, urinary, circulatory, respiratory.

Properties: carminative, nervine, antispasmodic, antiseptic, laxative, antilithic, analgesic, diaphoretic, anthelmintic, diuretic, emmenagogue, stimulant, alterative (root).

Indications: low appetite, flatulence, colic, constipation, abdominal pain, hiccup, dyspepsia, nausea, respiratory disorders, sinus congestion, cough, colds, fever, influenza, arthritis, gout, kidney and gallstones, dental pain, canker sores, parasites, fungal infections, chronic malabsorption, headache.

Precautions: high *pitta*, avoid during pregnancy (small amounts in cooking is ok).

Ajwan and ajmoda have very similar properties and can be used interchangeably in herbal medicine. The seeds have a strong aromatic fragrance and are used frequently in Indian cuisine for both flavor and to strengthen the digestion. They are commonly added to vegetables in the *brassica* family, such as cabbage, cauliflower, broccoli, and kale, as well as to heavy vegetables like potatoes to make them less *vata* provoking.

The seeds help to regulate the normal functions of *samana vayu* and *apana vayu*, thus promoting digestion, absorption, and assimilation, as well as elimination. Their warming and stimulating action kindles the digestive fire, burns *ama*, and increases the appetite. The whole plant of either variety is rich in vitamins and minerals, including vitamin C, phosphorus, iron, calcium, sodium, and magnesium.

They are pacifying to *vata*, due to their carminative (*anuloman*) and antispasmodic properties, and are used to dispel gas and relieve bloating, belching, hiccup, and colic. They also promote circulation and break up obstructions due to excess *kapha* and *ama* in the intestines and urinary and circulatory systems.

For slow, sluggish digestion the seeds can be taken as a tea, either alone or in combination with other warming herbs like asafoetida, ginger, black pepper, and *pippali*. They are calming to the mind and nervous system and can help with insomnia and for those who are prone to increased flatulence while sleeping. They are present in a number of Ayurvedic formulas, including *hingwastak* and *ajmodadi*, which are used to treat a variety of *vata* and *kapha* related digestive conditions.

A pinch of the powdered seeds can be added to a glass of buttermilk to improve digestion, as well as chewing 1/2 teaspoonful of the dry roasted seeds mixed with a little mineral rock salt after meals, especially when food is rich and oily.

Due to their decongestant action upon the lungs, ajwan seeds are also useful in the treatment of asthma, bronchitis, sinus congestion, pleurisy, and tuberculosis. They can be boiled in water with a little black tea and used as a steam inhalation to loosen congestion and relieve shortness of breath and sinus pressure. Taken along with equal parts cinnamon, they help in the treatment of colds and the flu. A good home remedy for acute pharyngitis, sore throat, and hoarseness of voice is to chew a pinch of the seeds with a pinch of mineral rock salt and 1 clove.

The root has alterative and diuretic properties, and is given in cases of generalized edema, colic, rheumatism, and liver and spleen related disorders. The powdered root also has a rejuvenating action upon the nerve tissue and is good in cases of general debility, mental fatigue, and weakness due to malnutrition. All parts of the plant are alkalizing, hence they are effective in the treatment of arthritis and gout. For this, even the juice of the fresh celery stalks can be used.

The oil extracted from the seeds can be applied topically to relieve achy muscles and arthritic joints. A *pinda* or herbal bolus can be made by tightly wrapping 1 cup each of the ground seeds and dried ginger powder in a square piece of thin cotton muslin, which can then be heated on a skillet until good and hot, and rubbed vigorously on sore and achy areas of the body.

To alleviate migraine headaches or sinus congestion, simply wrap a few pinches of the freshly ground herb in a thin piece of fabric and sniff as frequently as needed. Other uses of the seeds include amenorrhea, hysteria, parasites, fungal infections, and the prevention of kidney and gallstone formation.

ALOE VERA

Aloe spp.; Liliaceae
KUMARI

Effect on Doshas: Gel/juice: VPK- Powder (extremely cold): V+
Rasa: bitter, astringent, pungent, sweet **Virya: cooling** **Vipak: sweet**
Preparations: infusion, dried powder, gel or juice.
Dosage: dried powder, 250 mg–1 g; gel or juice, 15 to 30 ml.

Parts used: gel, whole leaf (fresh and dried).

Tissues: all tissues.

Systems: circulatory, digestive, reproductive, excretory.

Properties: alterative, bitter tonic, anti-inflammatory, laxative, purgative, rejuvenative, emmenagogue, vulnerary.

Indications: cuts, burns, fever, skin conditions, infections, conjunctivitis, constipation, bursitis, jaundice, hepatitis, enlarged spleen or liver, amenorrhea, dysmenorrhea, menopause, cystitis, vaginitis, cervical dysplasia, fibrocystic breasts, hemorrhoids, fissure/fistula, tumors, asthma, bronchitis, intestinal worms, ulcerative colitis, lipoma.

Precautions: pregnancy, profuse uterine bleeding, diabetes.

In Sanskrit, aloe vera is called *kumari*, which means virgin or young girl, because it is considered to bestow youthfulness, innocence, and feminine qualities. Aloe vera gel or juice nourishes all of the bodily tissues, pacifies all three *doshas*, and has a purifying and rejuvenating action upon the blood, liver, spleen, GI tract, and reproductive tissue. It has a cooling, softening, and soothing action, and is especially helpful for *pitta* related disorders of the plasma and blood, so it is often used for treating skin rashes, acne, rosacea, and other inflammatory conditions. One of the most common ways aloe gel is used in Ayurveda is as an *anupana*, or medium of intake, along with other herbs to enhance and guide their therapeutic effects.

In its powdered form, aloe is extremely cold and will deplete *agni* when used in excess, so it should not be taken for extended periods of time. As a purgative, it works to dispel excess bile from the liver and gallbladder. When taken as a tea, it can cause nausea and gripping of the intestines, so it is best used along with other herbs or in capsules for those sensitive to bitter taste.

The freshly extracted gel is a universal remedy to promote the healing of cuts, burns, scars, ulcers, and sunburns. Applying it to the eyelids is also helpful for various *pitta* related affections of the eyes, but the commercial juice bought at the store is usually preserved with ascorbic acid, which can burn the eyes.

Kumari also has a direct action upon the uterus and is considered to possess hormonal regulating properties. For uterine cramping, 2 Tbsp. of the gel can be mixed with a pinch of *trikatu* or black pepper and taken 2 times daily. Mixing 1 oz. of the gel with 1/4 tsp. *pippali* is also helpful for bronchitis. The fresh gel is slimy and soft, and a great remedy for dryness throughout the body.

Infants and young children can safely take 1 tsp. of the juice mixed in water once daily to nourish all bodily tissues, soothe the intestines, and promote healthy skin. This is also a good remedy for preventing and treating diaper rash as well as infantile eczema. For treating jaundice, mix 1 tsp. of the fresh juice with 1 tsp. *ghee* and put 5 drops in each nostril 2 times daily until the condition improves.

Keeping an aloe plant in the home is considered to attract wealth, as well as to ward off negative energies and spirits.

AMLA, AMALAKI

Emblica officinalis; Euphorbiaceae
EMBLIC MYROBALAN

Effect on doshas: VPK-
Rasa: all tastes except salty **Virya:** cooling **Vipak:** sweet
Preparations: decoction, infusion, herbal jam, medicated *ghee*.
Dosage: 1-30 g per day.

Parts used: fruit (fresh or dried).

Tissues: all bodily tissues.

Systems: digestive, circulatory, excretory, nervous, mind channel (*mano vaha srotas*).

Properties: rejuvenating tonic, refrigerant, anti-inflammatory, antacid, carminative, astringent, stomachic, hemostatic, aphrodisiac, laxative.

Indications: fermented digestion, tissue deficiency, debility, gastritis, colitis, ulcers, hemorrhoids, constipation, diarrhea, osteoporosis, biliousness, liver and spleen disorders, hair, premature graying, fever, gum disease, eye diseases, old age, mental weakness, eczema, psoriasis, heart disease, anemia, bronchitis, asthma, diabetes.

Precautions: acute diarrhea.

Amalaki is one of the best rejuvenating tonics known in Ayurveda, and is especially pacifying to *pitta*. It is also one of the richest sources of vitamin C and remains stable even after heating. It strengthens the immune system, enhances *ojas*, and nourishes all bodily tissues.

Sour taste, which is made up of the fire and earth elements, usually increases *pitta*, but this is not so in the case of Amalaki, due to its *prabhava*, or special potency. Its cooling quality helps to reduce excess heat and inflammation throughout the entire GI tract, so it is very helpful for treating conditions such as colitis, gastritis, hemorrhoids, and intestinal bleeding. It has an affinity to the liver, spleen, pancreas, lungs, eyes, and heart, and helps the body to better utilize calcium and regulate blood sugar.

Amalaki also nourishes the bones and promotes the growth and strength of hair, teeth, and nails, which are byproducts of the bone tissue. It can be used to treat *vata* conditions affecting the bone tissue like osteoporosis.

It supports liver function and is useful in the treatment of jaundice and hepatitis, as well as other *pitta* related conditions affecting the plasma and blood like hives, rashes, acne, eczema, and psoriasis.

It is a rich source of iron, which makes it a superb blood building tonic and very helpful in the treatment of anemia. It combines well with Western herbs that are considered blood tonics, such as nettle and red clover, to enhance their tonic properties.

Amalaki is one of three herbs, along with *haritaki* and *bibitaki*, that make up the famous *triphala* compound used to tone and cleanse the GI tract. *Triphala* helps to soften the stool and is used to relieve constipation. It can be taken on a regular basis without developing dependency.

Gargling with amalaki tea helps to improve the health of the gums, which makes it useful in cases of gingivitis and bleeding gums.

It also forms the base of the rejuvenating formula *Chyavanprash*, an herbal jam prepared in a base of fresh amalaki fruit along with other nourishing tonic herbs, which is one of the most revered *rasayanas* in Ayurvedic medicine, as it promotes strength, vigor, vitality, and longevity.

Arjuna

Terminalia arjuna; Combretaceae

Effect on Doshas: VPK-
Rasa: bitter, astringent **Virya: cooling** **Vipak: pungent**
Preparations: infusion (powder), medicated *ghee*, medicated wine, milk decoction with raw sugar cane.
Dosage: 1-6 g per day.

Parts used: bark.

Tissues: plasma, blood, muscle, fat, bone, nerve and marrow.

Systems: circulatory, respiratory, nervous, digestive, urinary.

Properties: cardiac tonic, stimulant, sedative, vasodilator, vulnerary, diuretic, hemostatic, digestive, analgesic.

Indications: heart disease, hypertension, hypotension, arteriosclerosis, congestive cardiac failure, angina pectoris, palpitation, bleeding disorders, high cholesterol, breathlessness, edema, poisonings, dysentery, hepatitis, sprue, diarrhea, internal and external ulcers, sores, diabetes, high blood sugar, anxiety, deep-seated grief and sadness.

Arjuna is commonly used as a cardiac tonic and vasodilator. It is balancing to all three doshas when used in moderation, although in excess it may provoke *vata*. It has the ability to either stimulate or calm down cardiac activity, depending on the body's needs. It is strengthening to the heart muscle, promotes circulation, and is effective for treating a wide variety of heart related disorders, arteriosclerosis, and high cholesterol.

Taken with warm milk, in doses from 3 to 12 g daily, *Arjuna ghee* can be used in breathlessness, angina pectoris, and congestive cardiac failure. A traditional medicated wine specific for the heart is *arjunar-*

ishta, which has a quick, stimulating action.

Arjuna has a mild diuretic action and is helpful in the treatment of cardiac edema. For this, it combines well with *punarnava*. Its astringent properties make it also useful in treating gastrointestinal ulcers, hemorrhage, bleeding disorders, diarrhea, dysentery, and sprue.

For peptic ulcer, add 1 tsp. of arjuna powder to a *lassi* (diluted fresh yogurt) and take after or between meals.

A general *tridoshic* formula for hypertension can be made with 4 parts arjuna to 3 parts hawthorne berries, 3 parts passionflower, 3 parts *punarnava*, 2 parts *guggulu*, and 1 part ground cardamom. This powdered mixture can be taken in 1 tsp. size doses in hot water, along with 1 tsp. raw honey, 3 times daily.

Arjuna has a stimulating action upon *kloma-agni*, the pancreatic fire; thus it helps to regulate blood sugar levels. For this, it combines well with herbs such as *neem*, turmeric, and *shardunika*.

For aiding the knitting of bone fractures, it can be prepared as a milk decoction or combined with other herbs like comfrey leaf or *manjista*.

Arjuna also acts on the heart chakra and is thought to increase *prema bhakti* (love and devotion). A nice formula to release unresolved emotions from the heart and lungs can be made by combining the powdered herb with equal parts *pushkaramula* (elecampane) and *brahmi* (gotu kola). This mixture can be taken in 1/2 tsp. size doses in hot water twice daily before meditation.

Asafoetida

Ferula asafoetida; Umbelliferae

HING OR HINGU

Effect on Doshas: V- P+ K-
Rasa: pungent Virya: heating Vipak: pungent
Preparations: paste, medicated oil.
Dosage: 100 mg-1 g

Parts used: gum/resin.

Tissues: plasma, blood, muscle, bone, nerve and marrow.

Systems: digestive, nervous, excretory, circulatory, respiratory.

Properties: carminative, stimulant, expectorant, antispasmodic, anthelmintic, aphrodisiac, antiseptic.

Indications: indigestion, intestinal distention and pain, flatulence, constipation, arthritis, rheumatism, epilepsy, convulsions, palpitations, worms, whooping cough, hysteria, paralysis, sciatica, earache.

Precautions: high fever, high *pitta*, hyperacidity, rashes, inflammatory conditions, urticaria, pregnancy.

Hing has anthelmintic properties and is used to rid the body of parasites and worms. It is also one of the best carminatives and digestive stimulants used in Ayurveda. It mitigates excess *vata* in the GI tract and helps to correct disturbances of *apana vayu*, the downward moving aspect of *vata*, therefore relieving flatulence, bloating, and abdominal discomfort. It regulates *samana vayu*, kindles *agni*, and burns *ama* in the intestines.

A small pinch of hing can be fried in *ghee* or cooking oil along with spices such as turmeric, cumin, and brown/black mustard seeds to aid in the digestion of legumes and counteract the *vata* aggravating effects of vegetables like cabbage, potatoes, and cauliflower.

It is also good for earaches and lightheadedness. A small pinch can be put onto a small flattened piece of cotton and wrapped to form a natural ear plug, which can then be inserted into the ear (not too far in) to relieve ear pain and ringing in the ear.

When applied locally as a paste, it is effective for treating ringworm and scorpion bites.

Because hing has a *tamasic* quality, it can be dulling to the mind. For this reason, it is often used along with lighter and more stimulating spices. The compound *hingwastak churna* consists of hing, ginger, *pippali*, cumin, black cumin, rock salt, and other herbs. It is used to improve the appetite and digestive power, and in many cases can be used where plain hing is indicated. *Hingwastak* is very effective for softening and breaking up impacted feces and other *ama* accumulations caused by improperly digested food, poor elimination, or unhealthy eating habits.

ASHOKA

Saraca indica; Leguminosae

Effect on Doshas: V+ PK-
Rasa: astringent, bitter Virya: cooling Vipak: sweet
Preparations: infusion (powder), decoction, medicated *ghee*, paste, medicated wine.
Dosage: 1-9 g per day.

Parts used: bark.

Tissues: plasma, blood, muscle, fat, reproductive.

Systems: circulatory, urinary, reproductive, nervous, respiratory.

Properties: astringent, sedative, analgesic, diuretic, stimulant, hemostatic, alterative, anti-inflammatory, uterine tonic.

Indications: bleeding disorders, hemorrhoids, dysmenorrhea, menorrhagia, leukorrhea, edema, fibroids, dysentery, morbid thirst, burning sensations, poisoning, uterine pain, endometriosis.

Precautions: high *vata*.

Ashoka has astringent action, is rich in tannins, and alleviates *pitta* and *kapha*. It helps to stop excess fluids from going out of the body, hence it is useful in bleeding disorders, diarrhea, leucorrhea, and menorrhagia. It has an affinity to *artava vaha srotas*, the female reproductive system, and helps to regulate the menstrual cycle. It is used to relieve uterine spasms, abdominal pain, uterine prolapse, and irregular menstruation. Having both a uterine sedative and stimulant effect on the endometrium and ovarian tissue, it is commonly used for treating uterine fibroids and ovarian cysts due to excess *kapha* and *ama* in the *mamsa* and *meda dhatus*. Arjuna has also shown to be valuable for the treatment of hemorrhoids, edema, and hemorrhagic dysentery.

Ashwagandha

Withania somnifera; Solanaceae

WINTER CHERRY

Effect on Doshas: V- P+ K-
Rasa: bitter, astringent, sweet **Virya:** hot **Vipak:** sweet
Preparations: infusion, decoction, paste, milk decoction, medicated oil or *ghee*.
Dosage: 3-9 g per day.

Parts used: roots and leaves.

Tissues: acts upon all tissues.

Systems: reproductive, nervous, respiratory.

Properties: rejuvenative, tonic, aphrodisiac, nervine, sedative, analgesic, anabolic, astringent, alterative, anti-inflammatory, immunomodulator, adaptogen.

Indications: fatigue, general debility, tissue deficiency, consumption, old age, senility, sciatica, insomnia, rheumatism, enlarged prostate, infertility, impotence, anxiety, multiple sclerosis, poor eyesight, boils, skin diseases, stress factors, overwork, heart conditions, paralysis, spermatorrhea, glandular swellings, difficult breathing, anemia, tuberculosis.

Precautions: high *pitta* and/or *ama* conditions, high doses during pregnancy.

In Sanskrit, *ashwagandha* means "the smell of a horse" due to the strong odor of the fresh root, which has a similar smell to that of horse urine. It is also considered to bestow the sexual vitality of a horse and is often used for infertility.

It is regarded as one of the best nutritive tonics for *vata*, but may increase *pitta* and *ama* in excess. It enhances the tone and strength of the muscles and nourishes the bone, marrow, and nervous tissue.

Ashwagandha is a good herb for increasing the quantity and quality of the reproductive tissue, as well as the blood supply and tone of the reproductive organs. It balances hormone levels and is considered one of the best male reproductive tonics, since it helps to relieve conditions such as spermatorrhea, impotence, premature ejaculation, and nocturnal emission. For enlarged prostate, it combines well with herbs like saw palmetto, *gokshura*, and *shilajit*.

It balances and regulates the immune system and replenishes energy from general stress, overwork, old age, or debilitating and wasting diseases such as cancer and tuberculosis. It calms and nourishes the mind and nervous system, so it is quite useful for treating insomnia and nervous tension, especially when taken as a hot tea or milk decoction just before going to sleep. It promotes clarity, concentration, and memory in the young and old alike.

Because of its *vata* pacifying effect on the muscles and nervous system, it is used in the treatment of rheumatism, neurosis, Parkinson's disease, muscular dystrophy, paralysis, multiple sclerosis, and the like. In neurological diseases, it often combines well with *atmagupta* (kapi kacchu), *vacha* (calamus), *bala*, and *saraswata churna*.

It is a good tonic for weakness during pregnancy in mild doses of 1/2 tsp. twice daily, as larger doses may cause uterine contractions. After childbirth, it can be used to stimulate the flow of breast milk and can be combined with equal parts *shatavari*, fennel, and licorice, and taken as a milk decoction or in hot water.

Due to its *sattwic* quality, ashwagandha has long been used by yogis to help increase and transform *shukra/arthava* tissue into *ojas*, thus promoting spiritual energy and enhancing meditative power. If there is no regular, active yogic practices, then it may just increase the sexual energy and desire.

Topically, a paste of the green root or fresh leaves can provide relief to scrofula, boils, and glandular or rheumatic swellings.

Other uses of this versatile herb include *vata* types of asthma characterized by wheezing and bronchial spasm, and hypertension associated with anxiety, nervousness, and fear. Furthermore, it is valuable in treating autoimmune diseases, cardiac weakness, anemia, and skin diseases such as eczema and psoriasis.

Avena

Avena sativa; Germinaceae

OAT, OAT STRAW

Effect on Doshas: VP- K+ in excess
Rasa: bitter, sweet **Virya:** cooling **Vipak:** sweet, heavy
Preparations: infusion, tincture.
Dosage: 3-9 g per day.

Parts used: milky seed pods, stalks.

Tissues: plasma, nerve and marrow, bone.

Systems: nervous, respiratory, circulatory, skeletal.

Properties: nervine, tonic, sedative, nutritive, antispasmodic.

Indications: weakness, stress, anxiety, asthma, incontinence, convalescence, old age, diseases of the nervous system, adrenal burnout, anger.

Avena is pacifying to *vata* and *pitta doshas* and is a nourishing tonic to the nervous system, adrenals, and heart. It helps to buffer the nerves from the stress and over stimulation of daily life that can eventually lead to depression, low vitality, and immunity. The unripened milky tops and green stalks are especially rich in silica, calcium, chromium, and magnesium, as well as B vitamins. Whenever there is exhaustion and a withering of vital energy, avena makes a nice addition to the overall treatment.

Its *vata* pacifying properties help to ease anxiety, restlessness, and nervous tension. For this, it combines well with *ashwagandha*, *bala*, wild yam, or *vidari*. It is quite effective for insomnia caused by high *vata*, combined with herbs like *ashwagandha*, *tagar, jatamansi*, or valerian.

For *pitta* individuals with the tendency toward irritability, anger, and to drive themselves too hard or to be argumentative, it combines well with equal parts gotu kola or skullcap to cool and calm the mind.

When increased *vata* pushes *pitta* into the nervous system, the hot, sharp, and penetrating qualities of *pitta* can burn the myelin sheath, such as in multiple sclerosis. In this case, avena may be combined with herbs like gotu kola, skullcap, *bala*, and *ashwagandha*. Avena is mucilaginous and protects and rejuvenates the nerve tissue.

As a digestive aid, it combines well with carminative herbs like chamomile, cardamom, fennel, and ginger. It is also helpful in the recovery from the abuse of amphetamines, coffee, tea, or nicotine.

An oat straw bath is a wonderful way to calm down *vata* conditions like neuralgia or nervous tension, as well as to soothe *pitta* related skin conditions like eczema and psoriasis. A simple way to prepare a very enjoyable bath is to boil 1/2 lb. of the coarsely shredded straw to 2-1/2 gallons of water, then add the decoction to the bath water along with 5 to 15 drops of lavender essential oil.

The oats that most of us are familiar with are the ones eaten for breakfast, and they are a good food for reducing high cholesterol and as a nourishing porridge during convalescence.

BAKUCHI

Psoralea corylifolia: Papilionaceae

Effect on Doshas: V- P+ (in excess) K-
Rasa: pungent, bitter **Virya:** heating **Vipak:** pungent
Preparations: decoction, paste, medicated oil and *ghee*.
Dosage: 3-9 g per day.

Parts used: leaves and seeds.

Tissues: plasma, blood, fat, reproductive.

Systems: circulatory, lymphatic, digestive, reproductive.

Properties: alterative, antibacterial, antifungal, antiseptic, anthelmintic, laxative, anti-histamine.

Indications: skin diseases (especially psoriasis and leukoderma), rashes, fungal infections, parasites, leprosy, vitiligo, menopause, blepharitis, scabies, ringworm, ear infections, bilious disorders.

Precautions: high *pitta* (in excess).

Bakuchi helps to maintain the health and tone of the skin and is used internally for a variety of skin conditions, such as vitiligo, leukoderma, psoriasis, and eczema. It is often formulated along with herbs like ***neem***, turmeric, ***manjista***, gentian, and ***kutki*** for these problems. Due to the strong connection between asthma and chronic cases of eczema and psoriasis, blood purifiers like bakuchi help to address the vitiated ***rakta dhatu*** (blood tissue) that lie at the root of these conditions.

It is also used to rid the body of parasites and all types of worms. For this, it combines well with herbs like *vidanga, shardunika,* black walnut, or wormwood. It is a time proven remedy for scabies when used topically, and is one of the most valuable herbs in the treatment of leprosy, for which it has been named ***kushtanashini***, which means "leprosy destroyer."

Bakuchi is a mild laxative, especially for bilious disorders, and is considered to posses hormonal like properties. It can help to support hormonal balance during menopause, in which case it can be combined with *shatavari, vidari,* or wild yam.

Bakuchi oil can be applied topically to relieve inflammation, burning, itching and fungal infections caused by disturbed *pitta dosha* in the general circulation and the skin. When applied lightly to the eyelashes, it helps to cure blepharitis, an *alochaka pitta* disorder. It is effective for anal itching due to intestinal worms, so it can be especially helpful in the case of pinworms in young children.

A couple of drops of the oil can be applied in the ear to resolve the discharge of pus of ear infections, or rubbed inside the ear to relieve itching or ringing. Other uses of the oil include massaging it on swollen gums and applying it on skin disorders like vitiligo and fungal infections of the skin or nails.

Bala

Sida cordifolia; Malvaceae

COUNTRY MALLOW

Effect on Doshas: VP- K+
Rasa: sweet, bitter Virya: cooling Vipak: sweet
Preparations: infusion, decoction, tincture, medicated oil and *ghee*, paste.
Dosage: 1-6 g per day.

Parts used: roots, leaves, seeds, stems.

Tissues: acts upon all tissues.

Properties: rejuvenative, antipyretic, alterative, analgesic, anticonvulsant, aphrodisiac, nervine, analgesic, astringent, stomachic, stimulant, cardiac tonic, mild laxative, vulnerary, demulcent, diuretic.

Indications: physical and mental debility, chronic fatigue, muscle atrophy, Parkinson's disease, spasms, cramps, tremors, stroke paralysis, Bell's palsy, low libido, nervous diseases, urinary disorders, bleeding, asthma, intermittent fever, sciatica, neuritis, menstrual disorders, asthma, cough, genital herpes, convalescence.

Precautions: high *kapha*, hypertension (best used in formulation).

In Sanskrit, *bala* means "strength." This herb is one of the best rejuvenative tonics for *vata* and *pitta*. Due to its heavy and oily qualities, it increases *kapha* when used in excess.

Bala nourishes and strengthens all bodily tissues, especially the plasma, muscle, nerve, marrow, and reproductive tissues, and helps to correct disorders relating to deficiency and weakness of the body and mind. It is commonly used in the treatment of chronic fatigue, general debility, wasting diseases, muscle atrophy, neurological diseases, as well as in convalescence and the elderly.

It helps to maintain normal muscle tone and coordination and to relieve cramping and neuromuscular pain. For this, it combines well with *vidari* or *ashwagandha*.

To relieve severe symptoms of *vata* in the muscle and nervous tissues, such as tremors and cogwheel rigidity as in Parkinson's disease, or clasp knife rigidity as in stroke paralysis, it combines well with herbs like kapi kacchu, *ashwagandha,* and the Ayurvedic compounds *yogaraj* or *mahayogaraj guggulu*. It is also one of the primary herbs used for hemiplegia and Bell's palsy.

Bala is unique in that it has both cardiac stimulant and tonic properties, thus increasing cardiac output with less risk of raising the blood pressure or heart rate. However, precaution should be taken if the individual is already experiencing hypertension or increased *kapha*.

Due to its tonifying action upon both male and female reproductive systems, bala helps to promote fertility and spermatogenesis. It regulates the menstrual cycle and is very useful in the treatment of menorrhagia, leucorrhea, and dysmenorrhea.

Bala contains small amounts of ephedrine alkaloids. It acts as a gentle bronchodilator in asthma and aids in relieving dry cough and bolstering weakened lung energy due to chronic upper respiratory disorders. It can also be used as an antipyretic (*jwarahara*) in deep seated and intermittent fevers.

It helps to mitigate *vata* in the bones, hence it is used in the treatment of osteoporosis. Likewise, it works on the joint spaces, another site prone to *vata* accumulation, which combined with its anti-inflammatory properties makes it valuable in the treatment of osteoarthritis.

Bala promotes mental energy and stability, and is a key herb for providing relief from daily stress and tension. Combined with other herbs that have an affinity to the mind, like skullcap, avena, *brahmi*, *jatamansi*, *shankapushpi*, and *ashwagandha*, it makes a great mental tonic (*medhya rasayana*) for the young and old alike.

Barberry

Berberis spp.; Berberidaceae

DARUHARIDRA

Effect on Doshas: V+ PK-
Rasa: bitter, pungent **Virya:** heating (*prabhava*) **Vipak:** pungent
Preparations: decoction, poultice, medicated *ghee*, paste, tincture.
Dosage: 1-6 g per day.

Parts used: root.

Tissues: plasma, blood, fat.

Systems: circulatory, digestive.

Properties: alterative, anthelmintic, bitter tonic, antibacterial, anti-inflammatory, mild laxative, antipyretic, amoebicidal.

Indications: liver or spleen enlargement, fevers (remittent and intermittent), skin eruptions, dysentery, jaundice, hepatitis, diabetes, gastroenteritis.

Precautions: high *vata* conditions, depletion of bodily tissues.

Barberry is a strong bitter that has an affinity to the plasma and blood, and is pacifying to *pitta* and *kapha*. It clears excess *pitta* from the liver, which makes it useful in the treatment of jaundice, hepatitis, and enlargement of the liver and spleen. It soothes the mucous membranes, burns toxins, and does *rakta shodhana*, or purification of the blood. It works well in treating skin eruptions like acne, boils, and rashes, as well as a wide variety of infections. It possesses similar properties to goldenseal and can be used as a good substitute for this endangered plant. Furthermore, it is less disturbing to the *agni* and the intestinal flora than goldenseal, especially when used for extended periods.

Due to its heating energy, it is less provoking to *vata* than most alterative herbs, which are typically cooling. It is also a mild laxative and is used to treat inflammatory arthritic and rheumatic complaints.

Barberry is useful in *kaphaja prameha* (type 2 diabetes) and is effective in controlling blood sugar levels and decreasing excessive *kapha*. A good remedy for reducing *ama* and body fat, as well as regulating blood sugar levels, is a mixture of 1 part barberry, 2 parts turmeric and 2 parts neem. Two "OO" capsules of this mixture can be taken 3 times daily with warm water after meals. The Indian variety of this plant is known as *daruharidra* and is similar to turmeric in action.

Bhringaraj

Eclipta alba; Compositae

Effect on Doshas: VPK-
Rasa: bitter, slightly pungent, astringent **Virya:** cooling **Vipak:** sweet
Preparations: paste, medicated oil or *ghee.*
Dosage: 1-6 g per day.

Parts used: aerial portions.

Tissues: plasma, blood, bone, nerve and marrow.

Systems: circulatory, digestive, nervous, respiratory.

Properties: alterative, tonic, digestive, nervine, hemostatic, antipyretic, laxative, purgative, diuretic.

Indications: alopecia, premature gray hair, cirrhosis, hepatitis, skin diseases, enlarged liver or spleen, anemia, mental disorders, dysentery, weakness of the bones, poor eyesight, loose teeth, poor memory, nervousness, anxiety, insomnia, nervous disorders, swollen glands, bronchial asthma.

Bhringaraj is pacifying to all *doshas* but is perhaps best known for its use in *pitta* related conditions. It helps to purge excess heat, bile, and toxins from the liver, gallbladder, and blood. It is used for hepatitis, cirrhosis, enlargement of the liver and spleen, skin diseases, bleeding disorders, and inflamed mucous membranes. Its action is quite similar to that of dandelion, although it is not as cold in action.

For the treatment of hepatitis A and B, it combines well with *kutki* (gentian), dandelion, milk thistle, or *shankapushpi*, I have also seen it work quite well in the management of hepatitis C.

Bhringaraj has an affinity to the bone and its related tissues, the teeth and hair. For strengthening these, it combines well with *amalaki*. It is known as *kesharaja*, or "king of the hair," and the oil can be rubbed daily on the scalp at bedtime to prevent hair loss, premature graying, and dandruff.

It has a *sattwic* quality that refreshes the mind and senses (especially the eyesight) and improves memory. Combined with herbs like *brahmi* (gotu kola), *jatamansi,* or skullcap, it calms, nourishes, and protects the nerve tissue. The oil can also be applied to the soles of the feet to promote sound sleep, which is a nice remedy for stress related headaches as well.

The paste can be used topically to treat swollen glands and chronic skin diseases. Furthermore, a poultice can be applied on a scorpion sting and the wound wrapped with gauze to draw out the poison.

BHUMYAMALAKI

Phyllanthus niruri; Euphorbiaceae

STONE-BREAKER, CHANCA PIEDRA

Effect on Doshas: V+ PK-
Rasa: bitter, astringent, sweet **Virya:** cooling **Vipak:** sweet
Preparations: powder, fresh juice, paste, infusion, decoction.
Dosage: 3-6 g per day.

Parts used: whole plant, leaves, root.

Tissues: plasma, blood, fat, reproductive.

Systems: digestive, urinary, genitourinary.

Properties: alterative, anti-inflammatory, antiviral, astringent, diuretic, laxative, bitter tonic, cholagogue, carminative, antipyretic, anthelmintic, lythotriptic, deobstruent, hepatoprotector, immunomodulator.

Indications: genitourinary diseases, jaundice, hepatitis, constipation, infection, ophthalmia, dyspepsia, dysentery, intermittent fever, diabetes, skin diseases, ulcers, gingivitis, scabies, gallstones, hyperacidity.

Precautions: high *vata*.

Bhumyamalaki is primarily used to clear excess heat from the blood, liver, and gallbladder (*ranjaka pitta*) and the GI tract (*pachaka pitta*). It is typically taken in teaspoon size doses in the early morning or evening before sleep as a mild *virechana* (purgative) to remove excess *pitta* and *ama*. It is very effective for jaundice, hepatitis, dysentery, and digestive complaints due to increased *pitta* and *kapha*. It helps to prevent the formation and accumulation of gallstones.

It pacifies *bhrajaka pitta* and makes a nice addition to the treatment of skin diseases and infections, boils, and abscesses. It also helps to relieve itching in cases of urticaria, psoriasis, and eczema. Here it combines well with herbs such as *bakuchi*, *manjista*, turmeric, or burdock seed. A paste of the plant made with rice water can promote the healing of ulcers, edematous swelling, scabies and other skin diseases.

As a cooling, astringent diuretic and deobstruent, it is used for flushing stones and urinary gravel from the urinary tract. It is also useful for edema, gonorrhea, and genitourinary diseases.

Mixed with *shardunika*, turmeric, or neem, it can regulate sugar levels and is valuable in the management of type 2 diabetes.

The tea or freshly extracted juice of the plant helps to treat hard to heal sores. Mixed with a gentle base oil, it can be used in ophthalmia by applying it around the eyes.

Bibhitaki

Terminalia belerica; Combretaceae

BELERIC MYROBALAN

Effect on Doshas: V+ (in excess) **PK-**
Rasa: astringent **Virya:** heating **Vipak:** sweet
Preparations: infusion, decoction, paste, eyewash, medicated *ghee*.
Dosage: 250 mg-6 g per day.

Parts used: fruit.

Tissues: plaśma, blood, bone.

Systems: respiratory, digestive, excretory, nervous.

Properties: laxative, astringent, tonic, rejuvenative, anthelmintic, antiseptic, lithotriptic, expectorant.

Indications: cough, cold, sore throat, bronchitis, laryngitis, catarrh, stones, chronic diarrhea, dysentery, eye diseases, constipation, headache, hemorrhoids, parasites, *kapha* disorders, liver and spleen disorders.

Precautions: high *vata*.

Bibhitaki is one of the three fruits of India's various myrobalan trees that, along with *amalaki* and *haritaki*, make up the famous compound *triphala*, which is used to treat a variety of eye disorders, such as glaucoma, poor eyesight and cataracts, as well as a host of digestive complaints (see *Triphala*).

Bibhitaki is a valuable *rasayana* for *kapha dosha*. It helps to control the water element in the body and is effective in preventing and treating congestive and accumulative disorders of the digestive, urinary, and respiratory tracts.

It helps to break down and expel obstructions in the *srotamsi* such as stones, phlegm, and impacted wastes and is also helpful in ridding the system of parasites and excess *ama*.

It is predominately astringent in taste and action, and it is unique in that it provides tone to the bowels while being a gentle yet effective laxative. It helps with the absorption of nutrients and promotes healthy bones and hair.

Its warming energy aids to kindle *agni*, the digestive fire, thus increasing the appetite without provoking *pitta*. It can be combined with *pippali* and mineral rock salt for sluggish digestion and poor appetite.

Bibhitaki is also useful in coughs and sore throat. For this, it can be mixed with turmeric and used as a gargle, or with *pippali* and honey for laryngitis or hoarseness of voice.

It improves vision and has a tonic action on the brain tissue, thus helping with mental functions.

It is antiseptic and can be applied topically as a paste to swellings and poisonous stings. As a tea, it can be used to wash and promote the healing of wounds and infections.

Bilva

Aegle marmelos; Rutaceae

BEAL TREE

Effect on Doshas: VPK=
Rasa: astringent, bitter, sweet **Virya:** heating **Vipak:** pungent
Preparations: decoction, jam, medicated oil.
Dosage: 1-12 g per day (dried herb).

Parts used: unripe fruit, leaves, roots, bark.

Tissues: plasma, blood, fat.

Systems: digestive, urinary.

Properties: digestive stimulant, anthelmintic, astringent, expectorant, antipyretic, anti-inflammatory.

Indications: dysentery, diarrhea, alternating constipation and diarrhea, parasites, Crohn's disease, ulcerative colitis, colic, gas, malabsorption, sprue, obesity, diabetes, edema, stomatitis, asthma, intermittent fever, depression.

Precautions: high *vata.*

The bilva tree can be found all over India, from the foothills of the Himalayas to the southern regions. It is considered sacred to both Buddhists and Hindus alike, and its leaves are commonly used in the worship of Lord Shiva and his consort Parvati.

The bilva fruit is a valuable medicine for the treatment of diarrhea, dyspepsia, and malabsorption. It works especially well for digestive disorders of the lower GI tract, such as irritable bowel syndrome, characterized by abdominal distention, gripping pain, flatulence, and alternating constipation and diarrhea. For this, it can be combined with equal parts *triphala*, licorice, and marshmallow. For amoebic dysentery and chronic diarrhea, it combines well with equal parts *kutaja*. Bilva is the leading herb in the semi solid jam *bilvadi lehyam*, which is used to treat chronic-diarrhea.

Bilva tonifies the colon and helps to improve absorption and elimination. It also binds the stool and burns *ama* in the GI tract, which may be essential in cases of diarrhea associated with *ama* (as in food poisoning or intestinal flu) or *krumi* (parasites). For treating parasites, it combines well with herbs like *vidanga*, *shardunika*, wormwood, or *neem*.

Being rich in pectin, tannin, and marmelosin, it promotes the healing of inflamed mucous membranes and intestinal ulcers. The regular use of bilva has shown to prevent bleeding disorders and piles. Used as a mouthwash, it heals ulcers of the mouth and gingivitis.

Bilva kindles *medha dhatu agni*, the fire element present in the fat tissue, and is mildly diuretic, so it can help to treat edema and obesity. Taking 1 tsp. of the powdered herb with warm water mixed 1 tsp. of raw honey first thing in the morning on an empty stomach can help to reduce body fat. A secondary effect of reducing *kapha* is that it can help with depression and melancholia.

When combined with equal parts turmeric and *neem*, bilva is effective in controlling blood sugar levels and can be useful in the management of adult onset diabetes.

Traditionally, a decoction of the leaves is used as an expectorant in cases of bronchial asthma. A decoction of both the leaves and the bark is effective in the treatment of intermittent fevers.

The fresh bilva fruit has mild laxative properties and shows some similarity to the herb rhubarb, which may be used as a substitute in certain cases.

Black Pepper

Piper nigrum; Piperaceae

MARICHA

Effect on Doshas: V- P+ K-
Rasa: pungent **Virya:** heating **Vipak:** pungent
Preparations: infusion, medicated wine (is one of the ingredients in *draksha arishta*), milk decoction, medicated *ghee*.
Dosage: 1-5 g per day.

Parts used: fruit.

Tissues: plasma, blood, fat, marrow and nerve.

Systems: digestive, respiratory, circulatory.

Properties: stimulant, expectorant, carminative, alterative, febrifuge, anthelmintic, antifungal, antibacterial, antispasmodic.

Indications: chronic indigestion, poor appetite, low metabolism, obesity, sinus congestion, toxins in the colon, fever, intermittent fever, cold extremities, urticaria, arthritis, epilepsy, warts, cystic acne, parasites, flatulence, colic.

Precautions: high *pitta*, inflammatory disorders of the GI tract.

In Sanskrit, *mara* means "that which destroys," and *icha*, "impurities." *Maricha* is one of the thousand names for the sun. This name is given to black pepper because of its extremely heating quality, which increases *tejas*, the fire element. It stimulates the appetite, promotes digestion, burns toxins, and reduces both *kapha* and *vata*. In excess, it may be drying to *vata*, therefore it is often combined with other herbs, including salt, in compounds used specifically for *vata* digestive disorders, such as *hingwashtak* or *lavanbhaskar churna*. To balance its drying quality, it can also be combined with moistening herbs like licorice or marshmallow root.

Black pepper is used to treat common colds, congestion, fever, sinus disorders, parasites, slow or variable digestion, colic, and flatulence. It aids the digestion of cold, raw, or heavy foods and drinks like milk, cucumbers, salads, or cheese. It also helps to decrease the *vata* provoking quality of beans, relieving flatulence, abdominal distention, and spasmodic pain. When used for short periods of time, it can be useful even for *sama pitta* conditions, as well as to improve liver functions. In such cases, it can be combined with bitter herbs like *guduchi*, burdock, or *neem* to balance its hot energy.

Along with ginger and *pippali*, black pepper is one of the ingredients in *trikatu*, which is one of the best formulas for stimulating digestion and circulation, eliminating excess *kapha*, regulating cholesterol levels, and strengthening the throat and lungs.

It promotes *agni*, which makes it especially useful when living on a light and *sattwic* diet. In ancient times, yogis and ascetics commonly lived on diets consisting of just fruits and roots. Since this kind of diet can provoke *vata*, they used heating spices like *maricha* and ginger, along with certain yogic practices, to maintain their inner fire. Nowadays, many people follow a raw or live food diet, which can aggravate *vata* over time. Here, too, warm spices such as black pepper can be very useful.

Topically, it is used to treat rashes like urticaria (*sheeta pitta*) by combining 1/2 tsp. of black pepper with 1 tsp. of *ghee*. This helps to calm *vata*, which is pushing *pitta* to the surface (and causing the eruption and itching). A traditional medicated oil called *marichadi tailam* is specifically used for treating *sheeta pitta*.

As a counter irritant, a very small amount of black pepper can be blown into the nose to divert seizures and free the movement of vital *prana*. As a medicated *ghee*, it helps to expel sinus congestion.

Boneset

Eupatorium perfoliatum; Compositae

Effect on Doshas: V+ PK-
Rasa: bitter, pungent **Virya:** cooling **Vipak:** pungent
Preparations: infusion, strong infusion as a laxative.
Dosage: 3-6 g per day (powder).

Parts used: aerial portions.

Tissues: plasma, blood, nerve and marrow.

Systems: hepatic, respiratory.

Properties: diaphoretic, antipyretic, antispasmodic, relaxant, mild laxative, purgative.

Indications: all types of fever, influenza, coughs, colds, congestion, aches, pains, chills, constipation, muscular rheumatism, indigestion, biliousness, jaundice.

Precautions: excessive use in high *vata* conditions.

Boneset is a cooling diaphoretic and is pacifying to both *pitta* and *kapha*. It is perhaps best known for its usefulness in treating the common cold and influenza through its ability to induce sweating during fever and lessen aches, pains, and chills. It can be taken as a warm infusion every half hour or so for such conditions. Boneset derives its name from its use in the treatment of a form of influenza that is accompanied by what was commonly referred to as a "break bone fever." It has shown to be quite effective during attacks of muscular rheumatism as well.

It can be administered as a cold infusion to clear excess *pitta* in the form of bile from the liver and gallbladder, and to purge *ama* from the entire gastrointestinal tract. In moderate doses, it acts a purgative to flush out toxins from the body during the later stages of the flu to promote a quicker recovery.

Boneset also helps to expel mucus from the upper respiratory tract and aids in digestive complaints of a *pitta* nature.

BRAHMI

Bacopa monniera; Scrophulariaceae

BACOPA

Effect on Doshas: VPK= (V+ in excess)
Rasa: sweet, bitter, slightly astringent **Virya:** heating (Prabhava) **Vipak:** sweet
Preparations: infusion, milk decoction, medicated *ghee*, paste, medicated oil, nasya.
Dosage: 3-6 g per day.

Parts used: aerial portions.

Tissues: acts upon all tissues.

Systems: nervous, circulatory, digestive.

Properties: nervine, alterative, rejuvenative, anti-inflammatory, antispasmodic, anticonvulsant, diuretic.

Indications: nervous disorders, mental disorders, epilepsy, senility, ADHD, Asperger's syndrome, autism, recovery from addictions, senility, rash, skin diseases, premature aging, diabetes, premature graying and hair loss, anger, headaches, migraines, irritability, adrenal insufficiency, stress, cystitis, colic, colitis.

Brahmi is another name for the Goddess Saraswati, and it refers to the feminine aspect of Brahman, the cosmic consciousness, that is associated with knowledge, learning, and the arts.

Brahmi is one of Ayurveda's most well respected rejuvenating tonics for the mind and nervous system. It is pacifying to all three *doshas* and kindles the flame of intelligence, or *sadhaka pitta*, in the brain. It may increase *vata* in excess, although this can be easily avoided if used in formulation with other *vata* pacifying herbs. It has a slightly heating energy, but its *prabhava* is such that it has a cooling effect on the whole system. Its regular use promotes cellular regeneration, thus slowing the aging process, and helps to sharpen the intellect, improve concentration and memory, and heighten consciousness.

As both a sedative and rejuvenating tonic for the nervous system, it helps to buffer and protect against adrenal burnout and general fatigue caused by stress and overwork. When combined with other *medhya rasayanas,* such as calamus (*vacha*), it improves speech and removes obstruction of *vata* in the mind and nervous system. Along with gotu kola, *shankapushpi*, *ashwagandha*, or avena, it calms and replenishes *majja dhatu* (nerve and marrow) and *manovaha srotas* (mind channel).

It is one of the most important herbs used in many neurological diseases and it can be effective in the treatment and management of Parkinson's disease, multiple sclerosis, epilepsy, ADHD, autism, dementia, and possibly Alzheimer's disease.

Brahmi is also useful in cases of depression and psychosis, for which *brahmi ghee nasya* is commonly administered and often supported with other forms of the herb, such as *brahmi rasayana* or *brahmi vati.* Another common use of *brahmi ghee* for psychological and neurological diseases in general is taking it internally. (See *Brahmi ghee*)

Brahmi has also shown to be beneficial in the treatment of skin diseases such as eczema, psoriasis, and even leprosy, as well as their associated emotional components. For this, it combines well with other *rakta shodhana* (blood cleansing) herbs like neem, *manjista,* turmeric, or burdock.

It pacifies *pitta* in the head and prevents early graying and hair fall when applied regularly as a medicated oil to the scalp. For this, it can also be taken internally along with herbs like aloe vera, horsetail, nettles, *bhringaraj*, or *amalaki*, which also have an affinity to the hair.

For headaches, especially migraines, it can be used along with herbs like *shatavari,* feverfew, gotu kola, ginko, peppermint, or skullcap.

Yogis consider brahmi to have *sattwic* qualities and to increase concentration and devotion. It is purifying to the *nadis* (subtle nerve pathways) and can enhance spiritual practices when taken regularly.

Brahmi's *prabhava* purifies both the lunar channel (*Ida*) and the solar channel (*Pingala*) of the subtle body, bringing balance to both feminine and masculine aspects. A nice meditation tea can be made by combining it with equal parts *vacha* (calamus) and a pinch of cardamom, taken in doses of 1/2 to 1 tsp. in a cup of hot water in the morning before practice. This tea facilitates the movement of *prana* into the central *nadi*, *shushumna*, and the ascending movement of the *Kundalini Shakti*.

Burdock

Arctium lappa; Compositae

Effect on Doshas: V+ (in excess, esp. the seeds) PK-
Rasa: bitter, sweet **Virya:** cooling **Vipak:** pungent
Preparations: decoction (root and seeds), infusion (powder or leaves), tincture, poultice.
Dosage: 3-9 g per day.

Parts used: root, seeds, leaves.

Tissues: plasma, blood.

Systems: lymphatic, circulatory, respiratory, digestive, urinary.

Properties: alterative, diuretic, bitter tonic, diaphoretic, antipyretic.

Indications: eczema, psoriasis, rashes, acne, liver diseases, fever, lymphatic congestion, nephritis, edema, hypertension (*pitta* type), gout, arthritis, indigestion (*pitta* type).

Precautions: low *agni*, high *vata*.

Both the seeds and the root of burdock are deeply cleansing to the liver, blood, and lymphatic system. It is valuable in the treatment of *pitta* related skin disorders, including stubborn acne, boils, eczema, and psoriasis. To deal with such conditions and relieve itching, it combines well with herbs like *neem*, *manjista*, barberry, or turmeric.

Burdock is also rich in minerals and vitamins, including iron, magnesium, manganese, and thiamine. Due to its secondary sweet taste, it is less *vata* provoking and reducing to the tissues than some other bitter herbs, providing that the person is not already weakened or depleted.

Burdock root is often found in the produce section of health food stores and Asian markets. It supports liver function, clears excess heat, and aids in digestion, which is especially good for *pitta* constitutions. It also makes a nice addition to a soup to relieve cold or influenza symptoms, and can be combined with other vegetables, ginger, and onion.

Burdock seeds are extremely bitter and cold, and have an affinity to the skin as well as to the respiratory tract. They are used in the treatment of skin diseases, throat infections, cold, influenza, and pneumonia, as well as in cases where both skin diseases and respiratory conditions are involved, such as psoriasis or eczema and asthma. It is worth noting that Ayurveda, Chinese medicine, and homeopathy have all observed the connection between skin and respiratory problems.

As a cooling diuretic, it helps to release excess *pitta*, support healthy kidney function, expel uric acid, and treat edema, gout, and psoriatic arthritis. The leaves make a nice addition to skin healing salves as well.

CALAMUS

Acorus calamus; Araceae

VACHA

Effect on Doshas: V- P+ K-
Rasa: pungent, bitter, astringent **Virya:** heating **Vipak:** pungent
Preparations: decoction, infusion, paste, milk decoction, smoking herb, medicated oil, *nasya*.
Dosage: powder, 1-6 g; tincture, 15-45 drops per day.

Parts used: rhizome.

Tissues: plasma, muscle, fat, marrow and nerve.

Systems: nervous, respiratory, circulatory, digestive.

Properties: expectorant, decongestant, stimulant, nervine, antispasmodic, emetic, carminative, *rasayana*.

Indications: colds, coughs, congestion, sinus headache, digestive weakness, arthritis, anxiety, memory loss, polyps, tinnitus, deafness, epilepsy, coma.

Precautions: high *pitta*, bleeding disorders, hemorrhoids.

Calamus is mainly used to treat *vata* and *kapha* related disorders. It restores the functional integrity of *prana vayu, sadhaka pitta*, and *tarpaka kapha*, hence it is a mental *rasayana* that promotes awareness, focus, clarity, and memory. It is one the most powerful rejuvenatives for the brain and nervous system, and is used to treat hysteria, neuralgia, nervous tension, hemiplegia, and epilepsy. It plays a leading role in the traditional compound *saraswata churna* that is used for many of these disorders.

Vacha oil may be used in *nasya* therapy for *vata* and *kapha* imbalances. Its *kapha* pacifying properties help to break up wet, cold, and boggy sinus congestion, and it is also effective in treating asthma, sinus headaches, seizures, loss of consciousness, and nasal polyps. As a purgative *nasya*, a small amount of the powdered herb is blown into the nostrils. This method is used mainly for increased *kapha*, although it can be quite intense and somewhat aggravating, and should be administered with caution.

The name *vacha* refers to speech, indicating its affinity to the throat region. It is indeed helpful for speech impediments, loss of speech due to stroke, difficulty in expressing oneself, as well as for stimulating low thyroid function.

As a digestive stimulant, it treats gas, bloating, abdominal discomfort, poor appetite, and excess mucus and *ama* in the stomach and intestines.

Applied as a paste on the forehead, it can help to alleviate headaches and when applied to the joints or the soles of the feet, it can soothe aches or neuralgic pain and is also useful for treating sciatica.

Pouring a few drops of warm vacha oil into the ear can help to balance the ether and air elements, which govern hearing, thus improving hearing problems, dissolving wax and eliminating ringing in the ears.

Although rarely a problem in small doses, its emetic properties can be counteracted by combining it with fennel seeds or ginger. Calamus is used in *vamana*, or therapeutic vomiting, mainly to expel excess *kapha dosha* and *ama* from the stomach and respiratory tract.

In the yogic tradition, vacha is considered purifying to the *nadis*, or subtle energy channels, and stimulate the awakening and upward movement of the *kundalini shakti*.

For medical use, a small amount of this herb can be added to marijuana (*cannabis*) to counteract some of its *vata* deranging effects.

Cardamom

Elettaria cardamomum; Zingiberaceae

ELA

Effect on Doshas: V- P+ (in excess) K-
Rasa: sweet, pungent **Virya:** heating **Vipak:** pungent
Preparations: infusion, powder, milk decoction.
Dosage: 250 mg-5 g per day.

Parts used: fruit, seeds.

Tissues: plasma, blood, marrow and nerve.

Systems: digestive, respiratory, circulatory, nervous.

Properties: stimulant, carminative, expectorant, stomachic, diaphoretic.

Indications: cough, cold, bronchitis, asthma, hoarseness of voice, indigestion, low appetite, poor absorption, poor circulation, nausea, belching, flatulence, colic, tooth decay, bad breath.

Precautions: ulcers, high *pitta*.

Cardamom is a highly aromatic and refreshing spice with a *sattwic* quality that helps to sharpen and refresh the mind and normalize the flow of the *pranas*. It is a gentle yet effective digestive stimulant. It helps to decrease *kapha* and *ama* in the stomach and lungs, and is present in a number of Ayurvedic compounds for this purpose. It is often added to traditional Indian milk sweets to help in the digestion of dairy and is a key ingredient in *masala chai* (Indian spiced tea) because of its flavor, digestive properties, and ability to counteract the *vata* provoking quality of black tea.

Cardamom has an affinity to the heart. It helps to stimulate *vyana vayu*, the aspect of *vata* governing circulation, and can be used to enhance herbal formulas for cardiac disorders.

A small pinch of cardamom can be added to a warm cup of milk and taken before bedtime to induce sound sleep. It can also be mixed with anise or fennel seeds and chewed before or after meals to stimulate the appetite, aid in digestion, and freshen the breath. I like to keep a few whole green pods in my pocket so I can chew one after meals.

It is one of the most effective medicines for increasing *agni* without aggravating *pitta*, unless used in excess. This is one of the reasons why it is used in formulas such as *avipatikara churna* and *trijata*.

To relieve a variety of digestive complaints, including nausea, upset stomach, indigestion, bloating, and hyperacidity, it combines well with herbs like mint, chamomile, and fennel.

Chewing the seeds also helps to improve the voice, for which it mixes well with licorice. Used regularly in this way, it is also a good preventative for tooth decay.

Cascara Sagrada

Rhamnus purshianus; Rhamnaceae

Effect on Doshas: V+ PK-
Rasa: bitter Virya: cooling Vipak: pungent
Preparations: decoction, infusion.
Dosage: 1.5-9 g per day.

Parts used: dried, aged bark.

Tissues: plasma, blood, fat.

Properties: laxative, bitter tonic, astringent, purgative (in larger doses), alterative, antibilious.

Indications: constipation, indigestion, enlargement of the liver, gallstones, dyspepsia, diabetes.

Precautions: high *vata* conditions, pregnancy, chronic diarrhea, *vata* type of hemorrhoids and *pitta* types that are actively bleeding.

Cascara sagrada stimulates *apana vayu*, the downward moving *vata* that governs eliminatory functions. It is a good herb to consider when there is chronic constipation with the need to keep things moving. Long-term use of this herb, as with most laxatives, will not necessarily correct the problem in and of itself, but it does have some tonic properties that can help to increase the overall strength of the colon when used with a holistic approach and in moderation. A *vata* pacifying diet and lifestyle is necessary for any chronic constipation disorders.

Cascara sagrada combines well with ginger and demulcent herbs like licorice or marshmallow root to help provide moisture to the GI tract. Many laxatives tend to cause abdominal discomfort and gripping.

Although the dried bark of cascara is quite gentle, it can be combined with ginger or fennel to ease as well as to enhance its action.

In Western herbalism, it is sometimes considered a bitter tonic that helps to simulate secretions in the upper GI tract. From an Ayurvedic perspective, cascara is not a tonic in the true sense of the word and would not be recommended for long-term use to strengthen *agni*.

Due to its ability to cleanse *ama* from the colon and improve its tone, it can be added in small amounts to herbal compounds to help enhance their digestion and absorption. It can be added to *triphala* for stubborn constipation, when *triphala* does not seem to be strong enough to get the bowels moving.

Chamomile

Matricaria chamomilla; Compositae

Effect on Doshas: V+ (in excess) PK-
Rasa: bitter, pungent **Virya:** cooling **Vipak:** pungent
Preparations: infusion, eyewash.
Dosage: 3-12 g per day.

Parts used: flowers, leaves.

Tissues: plasma, blood, muscle, marrow and nerve.

Systems: nervous, digestive.

Properties: antispasmodic, anti-inflammatory, laxative, nervine, analgesic, emmenagogue, carminative, sedative, emetic, diaphoretic.

Indications: stress, tension, muscular pain, menstrual cramping, teething, inflamed gums, sore throat, indigestion, peptic ulcers, digestive problems, headaches, conjunctivitis, dysmenorrhea, colic.

Precautions: can cause a (hay fever like) allergic reaction in some people; emetic in large doses; may increase *vata* in excess.

Chamomile is a gentle, relaxing herb to the mind and nervous system, and fairly *tridoshic* when used in moderation. It is helpful for *vata* and *pitta* complaints of the GI tract and is used for colic, flatulence, bilious headache, diarrhea, and gastritis. As a general digestive tea, it combines well with peppermint, licorice, ginger, or cardamom. It is quite effective in the healing of peptic ulcers, especially when aggravated by stress. For this, it combines well with herbs such as licorice root, marshmallow, *shatavari*, and *guduchi*.

For generalized stress, anxiety, restlessness, and even insomnia, it combines well with equal parts *ashwagandha*, skullcap, and *jatamansi*. It is an effective bedtime tea for energetic young children and their tired parents.

It is mildly analgesic and antispasmodic, and helps to ameliorate neuromuscular pain, headaches, teething pain, and menstrual cramping. It also has diaphoretic properties and is useful to relieve fever.

The essential oil of chamomile can be added to a warm tub or used to infuse massage oils to relieve sore muscles.

For conjunctivitis or any inflammation of the eyelids, a warm, wet tea bag or a cotton ball soaked in chamomile tea can be placed over the eyes. It has a cooling and cleansing effect, and helps to soothe the inflammation and draw out impurities rather quickly.

The tea can also be used to cleanse oily skin and has mild anti-microbial properties, thus helping to regenerate damaged tissues as in wounds, fungal infections, and skin ulcers.

In large doses, it can produce an allergic reaction similar to that of hay fever in some individuals, so people with a tendency for allergies should be cautious and use a mild infusion to begin with.

CHANDAN

Santalum album; Santalaceae

SANDALWOOD

Effect on Doshas: VPK-
Rasa: bitter, sweet, astringent Virya: cooling Vipak: sweet
Preparations: infusion, decoction, medicated oil, paste.
Dosage: 0.5-5 g per day.

Parts used: heartwood.

Tissues: plasma, blood, marrow and nerve, reproductive.

Systems: nervous, circulatory, digestive, urinary, reproductive, respiratory.

Properties: alterative, diuretic, sedative, stimulant, astringent, antiemetic, antipyretic, bitter tonic, antiviral, antibacterial, antihistaminic.

Indications: skin diseases, liver disorders, burning urination, dysmenorrhea, conjunctivitis, nausea, vomiting, hyperacidity, inflammatory conditions of the GI tract, cystitis, bronchitis, remittent fevers.

Sandalwood is perhaps one of the most sacred trees in India and China. The heartwood has an unforgettable fragrant smell and is used to make medicines, oils, incense, carvings of deities, and prayer beads. Its scent calms the mind and purifies the atmosphere. It is pacifying to all *doshas*, but is widely used for *pitta* related conditions. It helps to clear excess heat and toxins from the blood and liver, and to pacify *pitta* related emotions like anger, jealousy, and hatred.

Sandalwood oil (*chandan tailam*) is used for treating skin conditions such as eczema and psoriasis, and inflammation of the eyelids. In the case of conjunctivitis, the pure oil can be carefully applied to the eyelids with a Q-tip, but not directly into the eyes.

Eating a few drops of the oil with a little sugar can be useful for treating burning urination, cystitis, and to relieve nausea.

For dysmenorrhea, it combines well with herbs like *musta* (cypress), black cohosh, cramp bark, or *tagar*.

It can also be used as a dusting powder after massage and steam therapy to cool the body systemically or as a paste for topical application to inflamed, burning, or irritated tissues. It can be applied to the forehead as well to relieve headache, especially if caused by increased *pitta*. The paste can be made with water or goat's milk, if available.

Applying the essential oil of sandalwood to various vital sites, such as the temples, third eye, carotid artery, belly button, and on each wrist is a good general way to manage *pitta dosha*, especially in the summer.

For cleansing the skin, clearing acne and blemishes, and to improve the overall complexion, it combines well with turmeric in a ratio of 2 to 1. Deeply rooted pimples are a sign of excess *pitta* that has gone deep into the muscle tissue. To counteract this, *neem* can be added to the paste mentioned above to make it more effective.

A small amount of sandalwood can be added to formulas aimed at supporting the liver or blood, as it helps harmonize various herbs and enhance their actions.

RAKTA CHANDAN

Pterocarpus santalinus

RED SANDALWOOD

Red sandalwood has the same energetics as white sandalwood, but not the fragrance, and can be used in much the same way, although it is a stronger alterative and is often used as a paste for skin eruptions like boils.

For *pitta* related skin diseases like eczema or psoriasis, it combines well with herbs like *neem*, coriander, turmeric, and burdock.

Both varieties of sandalwood have a *sattwic* quality and are considered to calm and concentrate the mind. A paste applied to the third eye, known as *tilak*, is thought to awaken the spiritual energy.

Chitrak

Plumbago zeylanica; Plumbaginaceae

WHITE LEADWORT

Effect on Doshas: VPK-
Rasa: bitter, pungent **Virya:** hot **Vipak:** pungent
Preparations: infusion, decoction, paste.
Dosage: 250 mg-3 g per day.

Parts used: root.

Tissues: plasma, blood, muscle, fat.

Systems: digestive, circulatory, nervous, lymphatic.

Properties: carminative, digestive, cholagogue, tonic, hepatic, diaphoretic, stimulant, anthelmintic, antilithic, nervine, alterative, abortive, emmenagogue, catabolic, antiseptic, laxative, antibacterial.

Indications: anorexia, dyspepsia, gallstones, hepatitis, abdominal distension, flatulence, malabsorption, sprue, yeast infection, parasites, constipation, hemorrhoids, fissure, fistula, enlarged liver and spleen, obesity, scabies, ulcers, abscesses, lipoma, tumors, cysts, jaundice, anemia, bad breath, alcohol addiction, rheumatism, nervous diseases, diarrhea, high cholesterol.

Precautions: avoid during pregnancy, high *pitta* conditions, and tissue deficiency.

Chitrak is one of the best herbs to kindle *jathara agni*, the gastric fire, and *bhuta agni*, the digestive fire in the liver that transforms the 5 elements in food into usable elements for the body. It burns *ama* and is primarily used to pacify *vata* and *kapha*. It increases *pitta* and is one of the main herbs for *manda agni* (slow digestion) and *vishama agni* (variable digestion). It helps to improve the function of *samana vayu*, the aspect of *vata* centered in the small intestine that governs absorption and assimilation, and *apana vayu*, the downward moving *vata* responsible for elimination.

It is the main herb in the compounds *chitrakadi* and *ama pachak vati*, which are used to improve the appetite and digestive power, burn *ama*, relieve flatulence and intestinal discomfort, and treat hemorrhoids caused by increased *vata* or *kapha*, as well as to pacify *vata* in the GI tract during the fall and rainy seasons.

Chitrak does *lechana*, or scraping of fat tissue, while promoting fat metabolism and is good for treating obesity and decreasing tissue accumulations like cysts, tumors, gallstones and lipomas, all of which are due to excess *kapha*. To lower cholesterol levels or for congestive cardiac disorders, it combines well with *arjuna*.

A good general formula for weight loss or abnormal growths, such as tumors and cysts, consists in mixing 3 parts *chitrak*, 2 parts *kutki* or gentian, 2 parts *trikatu*, and 4 parts *punarnava* or dandelion. Half tsp. of this formula, in powdered form, can be taken in warm water with 1 tsp. of honey 3 times daily after meals. If cut herbs are used, then follow the standard decoction method.

Chitrak is very effective in the treatment of jaundice, congestion of the liver, enlarged spleen, dropsy and hepatitis, and is one of the main herbs in the *rasa rasayana* compound *arogya vardhini*, which is often used for such conditions.

Taken internally, it can help to rid the body of all kinds of parasites. Topically, the paste made from the root bark is used for scabies, ulcers, abscesses and other obstinate skin diseases.

Along with herbs like gotu kola, bacopa, and calamus, it has shown to be helpful in epilepsy, hysteria, and other nervous disorders.

In the case of rheumatic diseases, chitrak slows down the mobile quality of *vata* while burning *ama*, and is an important ingredient in *yogaraj guggulu* and *mahayogaraj guggulu*, which are used for treating certain kinds of arthritis as well as *vata* diseases of the nervous system. (See also *Guggulu Compounds*.)

CINNAMON

Cinnamomum zeylanicum; Lauraceae

TWAK OR DALCHINI

Effect on Doshas: V- P+ K-
Rasa: sweet, pungent, astringent Virya: heating Vipak: pungent
Preparations: powder, paste, infusion, decoction, oil.
Dosage: 1-3 g per day.

Parts used: bark, leaves.

Tissues: plasma, blood, muscle, marrow and nerve.

Systems: circulatory, digestive, respiratory, urinary.

Properties: stimulant, carminative, diaphoretic, expectorant, diuretic, aromatic, analgesic, mild astringent, antispasmodic, alterative.

Indications: colds, cough, influenza, fever, bronchitis, sinus congestion, dyspepsia, chronic diarrhea, flatulence, wheezing, poor circulation, cold extremities.

Precautions: high *pitta*.

This aromatic spice can be found in most, if not all kitchens. It helps to warm the body and is pacifying to both *vata* and *kapha*. It increases *agni* and stimulates *samana vayu*, thus promoting the digestions and absorption of nutrients in food and herbal medicines. It helps to decrease the heavy qualities of foods such as rice, potatoes, and dairy. It is similar to cayenne in its ability to increase *vyana vayu* (circulation), but due to its sweet *vipak*, or post digestive effect, is does not provoke *pitta* as much as cayenne does and can often be used as a gentler substitute.

It is used to treat colds, coughs, congestion, and the flu. It combines well with ginger tea during the first stages of a fever to promote sweating and to burn the *ama* triggering the fever.

As an expectorant for treating sinus or chest congestion, a mixture of cinnamon, ginger, and licorice can be made into a warm tea and sweeten with a little raw honey. This is also a nice remedy for sore throats. A pinch of this mixture can be sucked on as needed for a soothing effect.

Another good tea for treating a cold or flu in the initial stages can be made by brewing 1 quart of medium strength fresh ginger tea with a small stick of cinnamon, 1 tsp. of licorice root (powdered or chopped) and 1/4 tsp. ground cardamom. If there is a fever, then 1 tsp. of *tulsi* can be added to enhance its diaphoretic action.

It is one of the herbs in the compound *trijata* ("three aromatics"), which consists of equal parts cinnamon leaf (or bark), bay leaf, and cardamom, and is used to burn *ama* and strengthen *samana vayu*, thus promoting digestion and absorption. This compound is used similarly to the formula *trikatu* ("three pungents") to kindle *agni*, stimulate *prana*, and burn *ama*, but is less provoking to *pitta*.

Cinnamon oil or powder can be rubbed locally to relieve toothaches. As a paste applied to the lower back, it helps to relieve sore and achy muscles.

Cinnamon has a *sattwic* energy and is calming to *vata*, especially when combined with *ashwagandha* in a ratio of 1 to 4. It also helps to stimulate and refresh *kapha*, thus promoting clarity of mind, especially when mixed with calamus (*vacha*) in a ratio of 1 to 3.

Clove

Caryophyllus aromatica; Myrtaceae

LAVANGA

Effect on Doshas: V- P+ K-
Rasa: pungent **Virya:** heating **Vipak:** pungent
Preparations: infusion, decoction, powder, milk decoction.
Dosage: 1-3 g per day.

Parts used: dried flower buds.

Tissues: plasma, muscle, marrow and nerve, reproductive.

Systems: digestive, respiratory, nervous, reproductive, circulatory.

Properties: stimulant, expectorant, analgesic, aphrodisiac, carminative.

Indications: colds, cough, congestion, indigestion, asthma, bronchitis, laryngitis, pharyngitis, low blood pressure, impotence, hiccough, toothache, vomiting.

Precautions: high *pitta*, inflammatory conditions, hypertension.

Clove is an aromatic and stimulating spice that has a direct effect upon the digestive and respiratory tracts. It possesses hot, light, pungent, and oily qualities and helps to balance *vata* and *kapha*. As an expectorant, it aids in dispelling cold and wet qualities in the form of phlegm from the lungs and stomach. It is present in formulas such as *sitopaladi* and *talisadi*, which are often used specifically for this purpose.

It helps to improve the appetite and is effective for treating slow and variable digestion as well as indigestion. Like most hot, pungent spices, it promotes the digestion of heavy foods and can be added to rice dishes and soups.

A simple remedy for kindling *agni* and balancing *vata* and *kapha* is to garnish food with a little clove powder. It is one of the main ingredients in the warming Indian spice mixture *Garam Masala*, which usually also includes spices such as cinnamon, coriander, cayenne, and bay leaves.

A traditional formula containing clove, known as *lavangadi vati*, is used for cough, colds, congestion, bronchitis, and asthma.

The essential oil of clove or the medicated *ghee* prepared with clove can be used topically as a powerful analgesic for toothaches. For cavities, a small piece of cotton soaked in the oil can be placed on the tooth periodically until it can be filled.

A nice massage oil for rheumatic pain in the joints can be made by adding ten drops of the essential oil to 1 oz. of sesame oil. In *marma chikitsa* (energy point therapy), diluted clove oil can also be used to stimulate specific *marmas* for *kapha* and *vata* disorders. This works well on *nabhi marmas* in the navel region for digestive complaints, as well as *marmas* related to *prana vaha srotas* and *vyana vayu* (respiratory and cardiac points).

COLTSFOOT

Tussilago farfara; Compositae

Effect on Doshas: VPK-
Rasa: pungent, sweet, astringent **Virya:** cooling **Vipak:** pungent
Preparations: infusion, tincture, poultice, milk decoction.
Dosage: 3-9 g per day; tincture, 30-60 drops.

Parts used: leaves.

Tissues: plasma, nerve and marrow.

Properties: relaxing expectorant, antispasmodic, demulcent, diuretic.

Indications: coughs, whooping cough, bronchitis, sore throat, boils, abscess, cystitis, asthma, low lung energy, sinus infection, chronic emphysema.

Coltsfoot is a *tridoshic* expectorant and lung tonic. Its name literally means "cough dispeller." It has been long used in the Western herbal and folk traditions for a wide variety of respiratory complaints with much success, due to its antispasmodic and demulcent properties. It has proven useful in the treatment of conditions like common coughs, whooping cough, bronchitis, and even emphysema. It helps to dilate the bronchioles and dispels phlegm, especially when combined with herbs having a similar action.

For respiratory conditions characterized by yellowish or green sputum and sore throat, it combines well with other cooling herbs like mullein, horehound, licorice, and echinacea.

When there is more of a cold and damp condition, characterized by thick white or clear mucus, it is great along with elecampane, osha, ginger, or *kantakari*. Often a dynamic approach is necessary due to changes in the condition. If there is mixed symptoms, then heating and cooling expectorants can be formulated together.

Coltsfoot helps to make the cough more productive and relieves both the wheezy *vata* type of asthmatic conditions and the *kapha* type of asthma, characterized by profuse bronchial congestion and rumbling in the chest.

It is a *rasayana* that helps to strengthen and rejuvenate the lungs and *rasa dhatu*. For this purpose, it combines well with comfrey, elecampane, and *pippali*.

Smoking the leaves can relieve difficult breathing toward the end of stubborn upper respiratory infections.

A poultice of the fresh leaves can be used topically on boils and abscesses to draw out the infection. Here it combines well with herbs such as turmeric, red sandalwood, and onion.

Coriander

Coriandrum sativum; Umbelliferae

DHANYAKA

Effect on Doshas: VPK-
Rasa: bitter, pungent Virya: cold Vipak: pungent
Preparations: infusion, oil.
Dosage: 3-30 g per day.

Parts used: seeds and leaves (cilantro).

Tissues: plasma, blood.

Systems: digestive, urinary.

Properties: carminative, aromatic, diuretic, stimulant, diaphoretic.

Indications: allergies, rashes, burns, sunburn, cystitis, urinary tract infection, urticaria, nausea, vomiting, indigestion, boils, fever, hay fever.

Coriander is an effective medicine for *pitta* related complaints of the urinary and digestive tracts. It is a useful remedy for nausea, indigestion, diarrhea, and fever. A tea made from the seeds or the fresh juice of cilantro leaves, taken internally or used topically, can be very effective for hives and rashes, as it helps to pacify *pitta* in the blood and relieve itching. To prepare the fresh juice, blend a good handful of chopped cilantro leaves with just enough water to make it into a watery paste and run it through a fine strainer. It can be applied on the affected area and left to dry, repeating as needed. Wheat grass or Champion juicers are great for extracting juice from soft plants such as cilantro.

For managing a high fever, the fresh juice can be taken in doses of 1 to 3 tsp. three times daily, or as needed. In the case of fever in young children, mixing it into a little fruit juice or water can make it easier to swallow.

The tea and the juice are also helpful for seasonal allergies such as hay fever and combine well with herbs like nettle, *guduchi*, *amalaki*, and turmeric.

Coriander cleanses and pacifies *pitta* throughout the urinary tract, so it can relieve painful urination caused by urinary tract infections. For this, the tea can be taken in generous amounts throughout the day along with pure (unsweetened) cranberry juice nectar. Coriander tea is a good way to dilute this strong tasting juice and enhance its action.

Coriander is a common cooking spice and probably one of the best for *pitta* types. It helps to improve the digestion and absorption of food and is used in East Indian and Mexican cuisines to balance hot dishes by garnishing them with freshly chopped cilantro.

The seeds can be combined and toasted in a cast iron pan with other carminative spices like cumin, Ajwan, and fennel to make an after dinner digestive aid, especially for rich foods. (See *Kitchen Pharmacy*.)

Cramp Bark

Viburnum opulus: Caprifoliaceae

Effect on Doshas: V- K- P+ (in excess)
Rasa: bitter, astringent Virya: heating Vipak: pungent
Preparations: decoction, infusion, powder, tincture.
Dosage: 3-9 g per day; tincture, 30-60 drops.

Parts used: dried bark.

Tissues: plasma, blood, muscle, marrow and nerve.

Properties: nervine, sedative, antispasmodic, relaxant, astringent.

Indications: dysmenorrhea, menorrhagia, cramps, threatened miscarriage spasms, hysteria, neuralgia, TMJ, convulsions, nervousness, stress, *vata* and *kapha* types of asthma, menopausal bleeding.

Precautions: high *pitta*, low blood pressure.

Cramp bark is pacifying to both *vata* and *kapha* and helps to relieve muscular cramps and spasms. Having an affinity to the female reproductive organs, it is also used to treat premenstrual cramping, dysmenorrhea, menorrhagia, and scanty or irregular menstrual flow.

Its *vata* reducing action makes it useful in the treatment of nervous tension, neuralgia, hysteria, and flatulence. Its astringency can make it useful for treating *pitta* conditions like excessive blood loss during periods and/or menopause.

During pregnancy *vata* can easily get disturbed, especially from overwork or lifting heavy objects, which can cause premature labor or even miscarriage. Here cramp bark, along with herbs like black cohosh, *musta* (cypress), *ashoka,* and motherwort, can help to reduce *vata* and relax the uterus.

The antispasmodic properties of cramp bark extend to the lungs as well and can aid in the treatment of bronchial asthma. In this case, cramp bark may be combined with herbs such as elecampane, *pippali*, or *tulsi*.

A similar herb to cramp bark is black haw, which can be used interchangeably and has even a stronger action.

CUMIN

Cuminum cyminum; Umbelliferae

JIRAKA

Effect on Doshas: VPK-
Rasa: pungent, bitter Virya: cooling Vipak: pungent
Preparations: infusion, decoction, medicated *ghee*, medicated oil.
Dosage: 1-6 g per day.

Parts used: seeds.

Tissues: plasma, blood, fat.

Systems: digestive, alimentary, circulatory, urinary.

Properties: carminative, stimulant, diaphoretic, alterative, diuretic.

Indications: indigestion, colic, sprue syndrome, chronic fever, fatigue, nausea, vomiting, hemorrhoids, hiccup, chronic diarrhea, hoarseness, loss of appetite, skin disorders, urinary tract disorders.

Cumin is a common culinary spice with a long history as a medicinal herb in Ayurveda. It kindles the digestive fire without aggravating *pitta*, and helps to promote absorption and relieve intestinal gas. It is soothing to the throat, digestive, and urinary tracts and is useful in treating hoarseness, dyspepsia, diarrhea, urinary disorders, and gonorrhea

Cumin seeds can be very useful for relieving nausea during the first trimester of pregnancy by adding a 1/2 tsp. of the powdered seed to hot water along with a little squeeze of lime juice. After childbirth, an infusion of the seeds can be given to the mother to increase the flow of milk and alleviate *vata* dosha, for which it can be combined with fennel and *shatavari* in 1:1:2 ratio and sweetened with sugar.

Cumin seeds are commonly mixed with equal parts fennel and coriander seeds to create a tea that is great for improving overall digestive health as well as cleansing the entire urinary tract. Depending on the specific condition, other herbs can be added to this blend to enhance its effect. For example, in the case of poor appetite or weak digestion, herbs like ginger or cardamom can be added. For gas and bloating caused by *vata*, *ajwan* is a good addition. For hyperacidity and heartburn caused by *pitta*, licorice or peppermint are good choices. For slow metabolism and a tendency to gain weight, stimulating herbs like ginger, black pepper, or cayenne can be mixed in effectively.

A good home remedy for correcting diarrhea can be made by sprinkling 1/2 to 1 tsp. of roasted ground cumin seeds into 1 cup of diluted yogurt or fresh unsalted buttermilk.

A traditional *dhuman* (therapeutic smoking) recipe calls for smearing cumin seeds with *ghee* to be smoked in a pipe for the relief of chronic hiccup. Another home remedy is to apply the paste of the seeds to the abdomen to ease the pain and discomfort of intestinal worms and colic.

Echinacea

Echinacea angustifolia; Compositae

Effect on Doshas: V+ PK-
Rasa: bitter, pungent **Virya: cooling** **Vipak: pungent**
Preparations: infusion, decoction, tincture, wash.
Dosage: 1-9 g per day; tincture, 30-60 drops.

Parts used: whole plant.

Tissues: plasma, blood.

Systems: circulatory, lymphatic, respiratory.

Properties: alterative, antiviral, antibacterial, antiseptic, anti-inflammatory, diaphoretic, analgesic.

Indication: toxic blood conditions, blood poisoning, inflammations, boils, septicemia, upper respiratory infections, wounds, sinus inflammation, abscesses, chronic ulcers, gingivitis, gangrene, venereal disease, prostatitis, viral conditions, poisonous bites.

Precautions: high *vata*, dizziness.

Echinacea is perhaps the most widely used Western herb for stimulating the immune system. It is also used to treat viral infections and a variety of inflammatory conditions. As a first line of defense, it works well during the onset of a cold or flu and can be safely used by young children and the elderly alike. Because of its cold energy, it can aggravate *vata* when used for extended periods. If it is used for more than a few weeks, it is best to use it in formulation with other herbs.

It is very useful for *sama pitta* conditions, where excess *pitta* is associated with toxins and when targeting the lymph, plasma, and blood.

It protects the bodily tissues from the hot, sharp, and penetrating qualities of *pitta* present during infections, and helps to decrease *ama* and resolve pus formation.

Having an affinity to the lungs, echinacea can be useful during upper respiratory tract infections and combines well with common lung herbs like mullein, osha, elecampane, ginger, and *pippali*, as well as nutritive demulcents like licorice and coltsfoot. It is highly effective for sinus inflammation and infections and is often combined with goldenseal as a general anti-inflammatory and antibiotic.

Taken internally, as well as applied topically as a paste, tincture, or warm fomentation, it can help to reduce inflammation and pain from boils and abscesses, and promotes quick healing of septic wounds.

The diluted tincture or decoction can be used as a mouthwash to heal gingivitis. Here it combines well with herbs like *bilva*, prickly ash bark, bayberry root bark, and yerba mansa.

It is also an effective remedy for snakebites, especially in large doses. Here the tincture is convenient to carry and is fast acting.

ELECAMPANE

Inula spp.; Compositae

PUSHKARAMULA

Effect on Doshas: V- P+ K-
Rasa: pungent, bitter Virya: heating Vipak: pungent
Preparations: infusion, decoction, paste.
Dosage: 1-9 g per day.

Parts used: root and flowers.

Tissues: plasma, blood, muscle, fat, nerve.

Systems: respiratory, digestive, nervous.

Properties: expectorant, bronchodilator, antispasmodic, analgesic, mild diuretic, carminative, rejuvenative, analgesic.

Indications: colds, cough, asthma, cardiac asthma, pleurisy, dyspepsia, nervous debility, fever, muscle pain.

Precautions: high *pitta* conditions.

Elecampane is used in both Eastern and Western herbology as a lung tonic. In Ayurveda, it is considered to have an affinity to the heart and pericardium as well.

It is pacifying to both *kapha* and *vata*, and helps dispel phlegm and fluids from the lungs, making it is one of the best herbs in the treatment of pleurisy, pulmonary edema, and pulmonary tuberculosis, as well as asthma, wet cough, and chronic bronchitis. It has also proven useful to lower cholesterol levels.

For cardiac asthma, it can be combined with *kantakari* and *pippali*. In the case of pericarditis, it can be formulated with equal parts *arjuna* and *punarnava*. It also helps to relieve chest pain in the intercostal spaces caused by coughing or fractured ribs. Here it can be applied as a paste to the chest or as a warm fomentation.

Elecampane is helpful for replenishing *pranavaha srotas* weakened by reoccurring respiratory tract infections. For this, combine 3 parts elecampane with 2 parts each of *kantakari*, *pippali*, and licorice and take with warm water and an *anupana* of 1 tsp. raw honey twice daily. To help lower fever during the flu, prepare a warm infusion mixing it with equal parts ginger or *tulsi*.

Eucalyptus

Eucalyptus globulus; Myrtaceae

TAILAPATRA

Effect on Doshas: V- P+ (in excess) K-
Rasa: pungent **Virya:** heating **Vipak:** pungent
Preparations: infusion, wash, essential oil, *nasya*, liniment, steam inhalation.
Dosage: infusion of whole leaves, 3-9 g per day.

Parts used: aromatic young leaves.

Tissues: plasma, blood, muscle, fat.

Systems: respiratory, circulatory, digestive.

Properties: expectorant, antiseptic, stimulant, diaphoretic, rubefacient, diuretic, aromatic.

Indications: respiratory congestion, sinus infection, asthma, muscle aches, blood stagnation and lymphatic congestion, dyspepsia, infections, cuts and wounds, ulcers, gum diseases.

Precautions: pregnancy, high *pitta* (when used internally), kidney diseases. The older, less fragrant leaves can be slightly toxic and hard to digest, and should be used sparingly for internal use.

Eucalyptus has a warming energy and is pacifying to *kapha* and *vata*. Topically, it has somewhat of a cooling and refreshing effect on *pitta* when used in moderation.

Eucalyptus is valuable in cases of chronic and intermittent fevers and has proven useful in the treatment of malaria. Care should be taken when using eucalyptus internally due to certain moderately toxic constituents, including phellandrene and piperitone, which may irritate the GI tract and cause headaches and nausea.

The steam of an infusion of the leaves or essential oil of eucalyptus has long been used to open the bronchi and cleanse and disinfect the respiratory tract, making it effective for colds, flu, asthma, and upper respiratory and sinus infections. For asthma sufferers, I recommend using *eucalyptus radiata* rather than the *globulis* variety.

Drinking a mild infusion of the leaves in small amounts can help to purify the respiratory tract, stimulate mucosal secretions, and induce sweating. The diluted essential oil also makes a nice vapor rub during upper respiratory infections. Use 10-12 drops per ounce of base oil (jojoba or sesame) for adults and 5-6 drops for young children.

Furthermore, the essential oil can be used in Ayurvedic *marma* therapy on specific points that relate to the heart, lungs, and sinuses to free up blocked energy and stimulate the flow of *prana*.

Topically, a strong infusion of the leaves, which are antiseptic and astringent, can be used to cleanse mild to moderate wounds, ulcers, and sores. Similarly, the essential oil can be used in this manner when diluted with either water or a base oil, or made into a salve. Liniments and essential oil blends containing eucalyptus are useful for stimulating circulation and relieving arthritic or muscular pain and inflammation. A steam bath of eucalyptus is pacifying to *kapha* types and is refreshing to the mind and senses.

Eucalyptus also increases the appetite and aids in the digestion of rich, heavy foods.

For spongy and bleeding gums, the tea can be held in the mouth and swished several times a day. Chewing a piece of the leaf can provide a similar benefit.

It is also effective for parasites of the skin and has proven useful for treating scabies. Likewise, eucalyptus can be used to reduce fleas and ticks in dogs by adding several drops of the essential oil to their shampoo.

FENNEL

Foeniculum vulgare; Umbelliferae

SHATAPUSHPA

Effect on Doshas: VPK-
Rasa: sweet, pungent **Virya:** cooling (slightly) **Vipak:** sweet
Preparations: infusion, decoction, tincture, paste.
Dosage: 3-9 g per day.

Parts used: seeds.

Tissues: plasma, blood, muscle, nerve and marrow.

Systems: digestive, urinary, nervous.

Properties: carminative, diuretic, stomachic, stimulant, antispasmodic, galactagogue.

Indication: gas, bloating, abdominal pain, children's colic, digestive weakness, poor appetite, indigestion, urinary disorders, cystitis, scanty flow of breast milk, nausea, morning sickness.

Fennel has cooling and carminative properties, and is used to relieve excess *vata* and *pitta* in the GI tract. It is one of the best medicines to redirect *apana vayu*, the downward moving aspect of *vata*, thereby relieving flatulence, bloating, and abdominal discomfort. It helps to kindle *agni* without aggravating *pitta* and to eliminate metabolic waste products.

Fennel is a gentle and effective herb for improving digestion, especially in young children or those with chronic digestive weakness. Toasted fennel and cumin seeds mixed with a little rock salt and Indian rock candy can be chewed after meals to improve digestion.

Fennel tea is also a great home remedy for relieving nausea, which makes it quite effective for morning sickness. It is also used to promote the flow of breast milk in nursing mothers. For this, it combines well with *shatavari*, saffron, raw sugar, and cardamom. For treating colic in infants, fennel tea can be administered with a plastic baby medicine dropper, as needed.

Fennel is a *tridoshic* herb that is also useful to remove excess *kapha* in cases of bronchial congestion. For this, it can be mixed with ginger and licorice and taken as a warm tea with a little raw honey.

As a mild diuretic, it can be combined with coriander, *gokshura,* or *punarnava* to relieve difficult or burning urination.

It is commonly given along with purgatives such as senna or castor oil to diminish the gripping and discomfort often caused by their use. If stronger doses of purgative herbs are needed, ginger can also be added to synergize with fennel.

Fennel is a good cooking spice to counter the *pitta* provoking effects of hot pungent foods and spices. It is a great substitute for anise, its more heating relative used in *chai* tea recipes along with spices like ginger, clove, cardamom, and black pepper.

It has a *sattwic* quality that is refreshing to the mind and is also considered to be nourishing to the eyes.

Fenugreek

Trigonella foenum-graeceum; Leguminosae

METHI

Effect on Doshas: V- K- P+
Rasa: bitter, pungent, sweet Virya: heating Vipak: pungent
Preparations: infusion, decoction, paste, gruel.
Dosage: 1-9 g per day.

Parts used: seeds, leaves, tender shoots.

Tissues: plasma, blood, fat, marrow and nerve, reproductive.

Systems: digestive, respiratory, urinary, reproductive.

Properties: stimulant, demulcent, expectorant, rejuvenative, diuretic, nutritive tonic, aphrodisiac, galactagogue.

Indications: dyspepsia, dysentery, diabetes, diarrhea, loss of appetite, allergies, sinus congestion, chronic cough, bronchitis, influenza, dropsy, high cholesterol, neurasthenia, sciatica, arthritis, gout, convalescence, boils, carbuncles, enlargement of the liver and spleen, promotes lactation.

Precautions: pregnancy, high *pitta*.

The seeds and the fresh or dried leaves of fenugreek are common cooking spices and are a key ingredient in various Indian soups and recipes (like *sambar* and *toor dal*) for added flavor and to promote digestion.

Fenugreek kindles *agni*, promotes the assimilation of nutrients, and is pacifying to both *vata* and *kapha*. It is useful for treating digestive complaints such as sluggish digestion, constipation, flatulence, and abdominal discomfort. Its detoxifying properties make it valuable in the treatment of arthritis and gout.

Its highly mucilaginous nature makes it very effective in providing bulk to the stool and healing intestinal ulcers. For this, the seeds can be soaked in water and eaten as a gruel. To correct diarrhea, the seeds can be fried in *ghee* with anise or fennel seeds and a pinch of salt.

To reduce *kapha*, soak 1 heaping tsp. of the seeds in 1 cup of hot water, let it sit overnight, and drink the water first thing in the morning. This can be very beneficial to lower cholesterol and high blood sugar levels. In the treatment of adult onset diabetes, it combines well with herbs such as turmeric, neem, and barberry.

A tea made with the whole or powdered seeds and taken with a little raw honey can relieve sinus congestion. Another remedy for this is to sprinkle fenugreek powder on your food daily.

A paste of the ground seeds can be applied topically to help suppurate boils and carbuncles. For this, it can be combined with turmeric powder and fresh onion paste, warmed in a pan, applied to the affected area, and wrapped with gauze. It can also be applied as a hair tonic, as it is also considered to promote hair growth.

Fenugreek has a warming and stimulating action upon the male and female reproductive systems and is useful for low libido, impotence, leucorrhea, and dysmenorrhea. As a general tonic for *vata*, 1 Tbsp. of the powder can be boiled in milk and taken early in the morning. This is a good remedy to improve the health of the reproductive tissue as well as to promote lactation.

Feverfew

Chrysanthemum parthenium; Compositae

Effect of Doshas: V+ PK-
Rasa: sweet, bitter Virya: cooling Vipak: pungent
Preparations: infusion, cold infusion, tincture.
Dosage: 3-9 g per day; tincture, 30-60 drops.

Parts used: leaves and flowers.

Tissues: plasma, blood.

Properties: antipyretic, anti-inflammatory, vasodilator, relaxant, uterine stimulant, carminative, bitter tonic, purgative.

Indications: headache, colds, influenza, allergies, cough, difficult breathing, PMS, migraines, arthritis, insect bites, scanty menstrual flow.

Precautions: high *vata* conditions (when used in excess), pregnancy, using it along with anticoagulant drugs.

Feverfew is useful for relieving headaches, especially those caused by an increase of the hot, sharp, and penetrating qualities of *pitta dosha* in the *rasa* and *rakta dhatus* (plasma and blood), as is common in migraine headaches. It is also useful for headaches triggered by a strong reaction to chemical odors or synthetic perfumes, which is also a characteristic of high *pitta*.

It is a good relaxant herb for overdriven folks that have a great deal of stress and tension, and it combines nicely with herbs such as gotu kola or *tulsi*.

A tea of the leaves and flowers given along with honey is good for relieving coughs, bronchial wheezing, and symptoms related to common colds and the flu.

Feverfew is a mild uterine stimulant that can aid in cases of scanty menstrual flow, cramping, and other PMS related symptoms. It can be used as a digestive bitter and has also shown to be effective in relieving pain and inflammation during arthritic aggravations.

GINGER

Zingiber officinale; Zingiberaceae
SUNTHI (DRIED)
ARDRAKA (FRESH)

Effects on Doshas: V- P+ K-
Rasa: pungent, sweet Virya: heating Vipak: sweet (fresh), pungent (dried)
Preparations: infusion, decoction, powder, paste, fresh juice, candy.
Dosage: 0.5-3 g per day; tincture, 10-20 drops.

Parts used: rhizome.

Tissues: all tissues.

Systems: digestive, circulatory, respiratory, reproductive.

Properties: analgesic, stimulant, carminative, expectorant, diaphoretic, antibiotic, antiemetic, antibacterial, antifungal, anthelmintic, anti-inflammatory.

Indications: colds, influenza, wet cough, fever, indigestion, nausea, vomiting, parasites, candida, poor appetite, flatulence, arthritis, muscle cramps, menstrual cramps, high cholesterol, obesity, arteriosclerosis, heart disease.

Precautions: high *pitta*, inflammatory skin diseases, bleeding disorders.

Ginger is known as *vishwabhesaj* or "universal medicine." It has digestive, circulatory, stimulant, and carminative properties, and pacifies both *kapha* and *vata*. The dried root is considered to be more heating to the interior than the fresh root, which tends to act more toward the surface of the body and has a stronger diaphoretic action.

Drinking warm ginger tea or chewing a nickel size slice of the fresh root dipped in sea salt just before mealtimes helps to kindle the appetite, stimulate digestive secretions, and relieve flatulence and bloating. Cooking with ginger is a sure way to improve digestion and absorption. Since it is milder than other heating spices like garlic and chili, it is a good choice for those with *pitta* predominant constitutions, although it should still be used in moderation if *pitta* is high.

A traditional digestive preparation is made by combining 1 part of ginger powder and 6 parts of fresh ginger juice to make a paste that can be rolled into small pills that can be dried and eaten before or after meals.

Ginger has an affinity to the respiratory system and is a rejuvenating remedy for common colds, coughs, sore throats, and respiratory congestion. A general formula for head colds and sinus congestion consists of equal parts of powdered ginger, cinnamon, and fennel taken with warm water and raw honey. For relieving sore throat, combine 1 part each of ginger, licorice, and slippery elm (or marshmallow root) with 1/2 part cinnamon. This can be made into a tea by adding 1/2 to 1 tsp. of the mixture to 1 cup of hot water. A paste of the dried root can be applied to the forehead to relieve *kapha* related sinus pressure caused by congestion.

The fresh root is one of the best heating diaphoretic herbs used to promote sweating. A cup of hot ginger tea taken before bedtime works well to break a fever. For this, it combines well with *tulsi* and lemongrass. Taken internally, or applied as a fomentation, it helps to relieve pain caused by sore, stiff, and achy muscles. Even though ginger has a heating energy, it possesses special properties that greatly relieve generalized musculoskeletal pain and inflammation. According to modern research, ginger contains an anti-inflammatory compound called gingerol that significantly reduces muscle and joint inflammation. During an active flare up of *ama vata* (rheumatoid arthritis), and even in osteoarthritis, 1 to 2 tsp. of castor oil added to a cup of ginger tea can be taken at bedtime to burn *ama* and calm the hyper mobile quality of *vata* moving into the joint spaces. Ginger is often formulated with other anti-inflammatory herbs like turmeric and boswellia.

To maintain healthy cholesterol levels, a simple recipe can be made by combining 1 tsp. each of finely shredded fresh ginger, raw (shredded or finely chopped) garlic, and a little lime juice with a pinch of sea salt. This mixture can be eaten and washed down with warm water before or after meals, 2 times a day. This remedy tonifies the heart and lungs, and is also useful in cases of *vata* and *kapha* types of asthma. Since it is very heating, it should be avoided by *pitta* constitutions.

In the treatment of obesity, it is helpful to sip on a mild ginger tea with a little raw honey throughout the day to keep the *agni* strong and burn *ama* and fat. This is very effective when following a *kapha* soothing diet and lifestyle with plenty of exercise. Along with black pepper and *pippali*, ginger is one of three herbs in the Ayurvedic formula *trikatu*, which is also used to strengthen the metabolism and to treat *kapha* types of digestive disorders, obesity, poor circulation, and menstrual complaints. (See *Trikatu*)

A nice way to reduce ginger's hot quality is to blend a few slices of fresh, peeled ginger root with 1 cup or 2 of water and lime juice and sweeten with a little turbinado sugar. This delicious tea can be taken at room temperature or slightly chilled in warm weather.

Ginkgo

Ginkgo biloba; Ginkgoaceae

BALKUWARI

Effect on Doshas: V+ PK-
Rasa: bitter, astringent **Virya:** cooling **Vipak:** pungent
Preparations: infusion, decoction, tincture.
Dosage: 3-9 g per day; tincture, 30-60 drops.

Parts used: fruit, leaves, seeds.

Tissues: plasma, blood, muscle, fat.

Systems: circulatory, respiratory, urinary.

Properties: sedative, astringent, expectorant, anti-inflammatory, antioxidant, tonic, vasodilator, antidepressant.

Indications: memory loss, Alzheimer's, dizziness, dementia, tinnitus, ischemia, dizziness, vertigo, hypoxia, varicosity, multiple sclerosis, depression, tuberculosis, cough, wheezing, blood clots, stroke, mental exhaustion, fatigue, dysentery.

Precautions: bleeding disorders, if taking blood thinning drugs, in an over stimulated individual, high doses may cause headaches and tremors if *vata* is high.

Originally from Eastern China, the ginkgo is thought to be the oldest living tree species, dating back to the Jurassic Period. Chinese monks, considering it a sacred herb, helped to propagate the species in an effort to preserve it. Then it spread to Japan and from there was brought to Europe. Nowadays it exists almost exclusively in cultivation. It is considered a sacred tree both in China and Japan, and is associated with longevity. Both the seeds (nuts) and leaves are used in Traditional Chinese Medicine, while the leaves are mostly used in the West.

Ginkgo leaf is widely used for supporting mental functions by improving blood flow to the cerebral region. It is often used in the treatment of short- or long-term memory loss, Alzheimer's, hypoxia, strokes, dementia, vertigo, and tinnitus. It is mainly pacifying to *pitta* and *kapha*, and increases *vata* when used in excess, due to its bitter and astringent tastes and cooling energy. For *vata* conditions, it is best used in a well balanced formula containing heavier and more nourishing herbs, such as *bala* and *ashwagandha*, or the traditional compound *dashamula*.

It is also an effective heart tonic and vasodilator. It helps to strengthen the arterial walls and inhibits platelet aggregation that can often lead to clotting and obstruction. For this, it can be mixed with *arjuna*. For varicose veins it combines well with bilberry.

The powdered leaf is inhaled for asthma, ear, nose, and throat disorders like bronchitis and chronic rhinitis. Due to its antifungal and antibacterial qualities, the leaves can also be made into a plaster and applied to a wound.

A nice formula for mental rejuvenation consists in mixing equal parts ginkgo, *ashwagandha*, *brahmi*, and calamus with 1/2 part licorice. This mixture taken in 1 tsp. doses in a warm infusion twice daily helps to promote awareness, mental stamina, memory, and intelligence.

Another good way to use ginkgo leaf for the elderly, in their *vata* years of life, is to combine it with nourishing tonic herbs like *ashwagandha, kapikacchu*, or *bala*.

Ginkgo seeds (nuts) are a revitalizing *rasayana*. They contain antioxidant properties that help to protect the cells and promote longevity. In Chinese Medicine they are known to have bronchial dilating properties and help to expectorate mucus from the chest, stop wheezing and coughs, and aid in the treatment of tuberculosis and certain urinary tract disorders.

The seeds can also be eaten to promote digestion. They help to suppress the effects of wine and to recover from illnesses. They are considered a kidney tonic and increase sexual energy. The cooked seeds help to stabilize the production of sperm and the raw seeds are said to have anti-cancer properties.

GOKSHURA

Tribulis terrestris; Zygophyllcaceae

CALTROPS

Effect on Doshas: VPK=
Rasa: sweet, bitter **Virya:** cooling **Vipak:** sweet
Preparations: infusion, decoction, medicated oil.
Dosage: 1-9 g per day.

Parts used: fruit.

Tissues: plasma, blood, fat, marrow and nerve, reproductive.

Systems: urinary, reproductive, nervous, respiratory, circulatory, digestive.

Properties: diuretic, demulcent, lithotriptic, aphrodisiac, analgesic, nervine, tonic, rejuvenative, antispasmodic, alterative.

Indications: painful or difficult urination, kidney or bladder stones, edema, cystitis, nephritis, hematuria, gout, high cholesterol, rheumatism, lumbago, hemorrhoids, impotence, infertility, seminal debility, venereal disease, sciatica, cough, dyspnea, diabetes, enlarged prostate.

Precautions: dehydration (in excess).

Gokshura is rejuvenating as well as cleansing to the genitourinary tract. It balances all three *doshas*. It is a cooling diuretic and demulcent herb commonly used for painful urination, urinary tract infections (both acute and chronic), urinary stones, prostate problems, and a variety of kidney related diseases. Unlike some diuretics that tend to weaken the system when taken on a regular basis, gokshura strengthens and revitalizes it.

Gokshura also enhances the tone of the reproductive organs in both men and women, especially when taken as a milk decoction. For impotence or spermaturia, it can be prepared as a milk decoction with equal parts *ashwagandha* and sweetened with raw honey.

It has shown to be of value for problems such as heart disease, high cholesterol, and fatty infiltration of the liver. For such conditions, *gokshuradi guggulu*, which is used when a stronger effect of *gokshura* is needed, can be an effective component to a well rounded treatment plan.

Gokshura is also beneficial in the treatment of hypertension when combined with herbs like *punarnava*, *arjuna*, hawthorne, and passionflower.

It helps to rid the system of nitrogenous wastes, hence it is a reliable remedy for the treatment of gout and rheumatism. For this, it can be used with herbs such as nettles, *ajwan*, celery seeds, *punarnava,* and *kaishore* or *rasnadi guggulu*.

When mixed with equal parts *neem* and turmeric, it works well to balance blood sugar levels and increase pancreatic function.

For urinary tract infections, it combines well with herbs like *shatavari*, *punarnava*, coriander, uva ursi, or pipsissewa. A useful remedy for kidney stones can be made with equal parts gokshura, *punarnava*, gravel root, coriander, corn silk, and marshmallow root.

Goldenseal

Hydrastis canadensis; Ranunculaceae

Effect on Doshas: V+ PK-
Rasa: bitter, astringent **Virya:** cooling **Vipak:** pungent
Preparations: decoction, infusion, tincture, eyewash, paste, poultice.
Dosage: powder, 3-6 g per day; tincture, 30-40 drops 2-5 times per day.

Parts used: roots.

Tissues: plasma, blood, muscle, fat.

Systems: digestive, circulatory, lymphatic.

Properties: alterative, antibiotic, antiseptic, anti-inflammatory, bitter tonic, astringent, hemostatic, antipyretic, diuretic, laxative, anthelmintic.

Indications: hepatitis, jaundice, rashes, infectious diseases, chronic infections, gastritis, hemorrhoids, bleeding, ulcers, influenza, fever, sinus congestion, malaria, lymphatic and glandular swelling, inflamed eyes, amebic dysentery, heartburn, biliousness, leucorrhea, menorrhagia, vaginal yeast infections.

Precautions: high *vata*, dizziness, pregnancy, tissue depletion, debility due to illness.

Goldenseal is one of the strongest Western herbs used to treat inflammation associated with both acute and chronic infections. It has an extremely cold and cleansing action, which quickly clears excess *pitta* and toxins from the blood, liver, spleen, lymphatic system, skin, and GI tract. It also removes excessive dampness associated with *bodhaka kapha* present in the head, especially the sinus cavities, as well as *avalambak kapha* in the lungs. Here it reduces nasal catarrh and inflammation brought on by the common cold or seasonal and environmental allergies.

In both *kapha* and *pitta* related gynecological conditions, including vaginal yeast infection, leucorrhea, and menorrhagia, it helps to clear and purify the mucous membranes, dry up abnormal discharges, and check excess bleeding.

Goldenseal is also useful in the case of intestinal inflammation, hyperacidity, or *amla pitta* (sour stomach), which is a *sama pitta* condition that can lead to fermentation, stagnation, and gastric reflux. Here it can be used along with other *pitta* balancing herbs like *amalaki* and *guduchi*, as well as the Ayurvedic compound *avipattikara churna*. A similar Western herbal compound used such conditions is Neutralizing Cordial, which contains goldenseal along with Ceylon cinnamon, rhubarb, and peppermint spirits. Both of these compounds contain cooling herbs to balance and purge excess *pitta* and *ama*, along with warming herbs to support the digestive energy and burn toxins. Goldenseal also helps to improve the flow of bile and aids in the digestion of fats.

Its powerful antibiotic action fights deep-seated infections, including chronic tooth abscess, systemic staphylococcal infections, and repeated boils where *pitta* has penetrated into *mamsa dhatu* (muscle tissue). The tea or paste makes a good topical antiseptic wash or poultice for wounds. The well-strained tea makes a good eyewash for eye inflammation and infections, including conjunctivitis and blepharitis.

When *pitta* from the liver is pushed toward the colon, it can cause inflammation in that area as well as *pitta* type of hemorrhoids, characterized by pain, itching, and bleeding. In this case, goldenseal combines well with herbs like *neem*, barberry, aloe vera, *guggulu*, and *guduchi*.

Goldenseal is also a good remedy to combat influenza and fevers. For low grade and protracted fevers, it is best used with warm diaphoretics such as *tulsi*, black pepper, or fresh ginger to burn *ama* and unblock the sweat channels. For high fevers, it can be combined with cold diaphoretic or antipyretic herbs like yarrow, boneset, *neem*, or *maha sudarshan*.

Goldenseal should be used with care, especially by *vata* types, because it provokes the cold, dry, and light qualities of *vata dosha*, weakens the digestive fire, and can destroy beneficial intestinal flora. However, it is not nearly as harsh on the intestinal tract as conventional antibiotic drugs, especially when used in moderation and along with plenty of fluids to help the organs with the elimination of toxins, particularly the liver and kidneys. It is best taken in doses of 1/2 tsp. or two "00" size capsules 2-3 times daily. It can have a gentler action when used in combination with other herbs, so I would typically mix it with either ginger or cinnamon for extended use.

Gotu Kola

Centella/Hydrocotyle asiatica; Umbelliferae

MANDUKAPARNI / BRAHMI

Effect on Doshas: VPK=
Rasa: bitter, sweet, astringent Virya: cooling Vipak: sweet
Preparations: infusion, milk decoction, medicated *ghee*, paste, medicated oil, *nasya*.
Dosage: 3-30 g per day.

Parts used: aerial portions.

Tissues: plasma, blood, muscle, bone marrow and nerve.

Systems: nervous, circulatory, digestive.

Properties: nervine, alterative, rejuvenative, diuretic, febrifuge, antispasmodic.

Indications: nervous disorders, mental disorders, epilepsy, senility, rashes, skin diseases, venereal diseases, premature aging, diabetes, hypoglycemia, epilepsy, premature graying and hair loss, anger, irritability, adrenal insufficiency, poor immunity, stress, colitis.

There is often a discrepancy as to whether gotu kola should be referred to as *brahmi* or not, since the *brahmi* most commonly used in Ayurveda is *bacopa monniera*. Another native plant of India that is referred to as *brahmi* is *hydrocotyle asiatica*, which is a variety of gotu kola also known as *mandukaparni*. The variety of gotu kola most commonly used in the West is *centella asiatica*. In fact, these herbs share very similar properties and energetics, although *bacopa monniera* is stronger in action and can increase *vata* in excess, which can be easily balanced when used in formulation.

Gotu kola is an excellent rejuvenative tonic for the mind and nervous system that promotes cellular regeneration and slows the aging process. It rejuvenates and pacifies all three *doshas* and helps to improve speech, memory, awareness, and intelligence, which make it useful to treat a wide variety of psychological and neurological disorders. It is also supportive to the immune system and adrenal glands, and helps to effectively treat intermittent or periodic fevers like malaria.

It supports proper functions of the liver, spleen, and pancreas and is a great blood purifier used in chronic skin diseases like psoriasis, eczema, and leprosy. It kindles and regulates *kloma-agni* (the pancreatic fire) and is also helpful in treating hypoglycemia and diabetes. The paste or medicated *ghee* can be applied topically to relieve swelling, inflammation, and itching.

Like *brahmi* oil, gotu kola oil is often used to combat stress and promote sound sleep, as well as for preventing early graying and hair loss. Applying it to the scalp and the soles of the feet before bedtime is a nice addition to a daily routine. For *pitta* types, gotu kola oil prepared with coconut oil is better over that with sesame oil, which has a warmer action, although both are generally considered *tridoshic*.

The medicated *ghee* (similar to *brahmi ghee*) helps to nourish and protect the mind and nervous system, and is also used in the treatment of headaches, depression, and mental lethargy, as well as conditions like multiple sclerosis and ulcerative colitis. When administered as a *nasya* (nasal therapy), use 2 to 5 drops in each nostril on an empty stomach twice a day. Taken internally, the dosage would be 1-3 tsp. in a cup of warm milk or water 2 times daily.

Gotu kola has the ability to enhance *sattwic* qualities in the mind and purify the *nadis* (subtle nerve channels), thus being a valuable herb for spiritual practices like yoga and meditation. Combined with equal parts *vacha*, it makes a good tea to promote concentration and meditation. Gotu kola is cooling, harmonizing, and purifying to the lunar *nadi* known as *Ida*, whereas *vacha* is heating and purifies the solar channel *Pingala*. One of the goals of hatha yoga is to balance these two channels to help promote the flow of spiritual energy into the central *nadi Shushumna*.

Gravel Root

Eupatorium purpureum; Compositae

Effect on Doshas: V+ PK –
Rasa: bitter, pungent Virya: cooling Vipak: pungent
Preparations: tincture, infusion, decoction.
Dosage: 3-9 g per day; tincture, 30-90 drops.

Parts used: rhizome (root), leaves, flowers.

Tissues: plasma, blood, nerve and marrow.

Systems: circulatory, urinary, nervous.

Properties: diuretic, lithotriptic, nervine, astringent, relaxant, tonic.

Indications: chronic renal disorders, hematuria, dropsy, gonorrhea, kidney stones, gravel, chronic cystitis, rheumatism, prostate disorders, Bright's disease, diabetes, weakness of the pelvic organs.

Precautions: high *vata*.

Gravel root is a cooling diuretic and lithotriptic that is useful in treating excess *pitta* and *kapha* conditions of the kidneys, ureters, and bladder. It brings tone to the pelvic viscera and mucous membranes, and helps to break down and flush out stones and renal calculi in *mutra vahasrotas* (the urinary system). For this, it works well by itself or along with other diuretic herbs that potentiate its action, such as *punarnava, gokshura, manjista*, dandelion leaf, or cornsilk. Demulcent herbs like marshmallow or licorice root can help to ease the passing of stones and are a nice addition to a kidney formula.

The tea made from the leaves and root is also used for treating cystitis, urethritis, hematuria, strangury, incontinence in children, and impotence. It is useful in cases of gout and rheumatism, as it promotes the removal of wastes from the kidneys.

For benign prostatic hyperplasia (enlarged prostate), gravel root combines well with herbs such as *ashwagandha, punarnava,* kapi kacchu, *gokshura, shilajit*, and saw palmetto.

To balance its *vata* provoking qualities, it can be mixed with heating diuretics like *ajwan*, parsley, or juniper berries.

GUDUCHI

Tinospora cordifolia; Menispermaceae

Effect on Doshas: VPK=
Rasa: bitter, pungent, slightly sweet and astringent **Virya:** warming **Vipak:** sweet
Preparations: infusion, decoction, medicated *ghee*, *sattwa* (starchy extract).
Dosage: 3-15 g per day.

Parts used: whole plant.

Tissues: plasma, blood, fat, reproductive.

Systems: digestive, reproductive, immune, urinary.

Properties: anti-inflammatory, antibiotic, antipyretic, alterative, diuretic, bitter tonic, aphrodisiac, tonic.

Indications: fever, burning sensations, liver disease, high cholesterol, constipation, digestive disorders, edema, kidney and gallstones, diabetes, prostate disorders, impotence, kidney diseases, gout, skin diseases, rashes, viral infections, bacterial infections, arthritis, hemorrhoids.

Guduchi pacifies all three *doshas*, although it is best known for treating almost any kind of *pitta* disorder since it balances and regulates all *pitta* subtypes in the body.

It contains berberine and other alkaloids that help to neutralize and burn *ama*. It is used to lower fevers, especially when chronic or intermittent, as in the case of malaria or autoimmune diseases. It is a good addition to cold and flu formulas to support the body's immunity. Simply taking guduchi by itself can help those who are very susceptible to getting sick during the winter months or who suffer from seasonal or environmental allergies. It is also valuable in the treatment of liver and spleen disorders, burning sensations, skin diseases, infections, and headache.

Due to its bitter yet heating properties, it kindles *jathara agni*, the digestive fire, without aggravating *pitta* and is helpful in the treatment of digestive disorders like dysentery, colitis, Crohn's disease, gastric reflux, and irritable bowel syndrome with alternating constipation and diarrhea.

Guduchi protects and rejuvenates the liver and is quite useful for treating hepatitis, cirrhosis, and toxic effects of drugs and chemicals. For this, it combines well with other blood cleansing herbs like *neem, kutki, shankapushpi,* and milk thistle. It is also useful for stubborn chronic skin conditions such as psoriasis, eczema, boils, and acne.

The fresh plant is considered to have a stronger diuretic action than the dried herb, although the dried herb can be used effectively to relieve inflammation and remove toxins via the urinary system (*mutra vahasrotas)*, and is also helpful in the treatment of arthritis and gout.

Guduchi helps to protect *ojas* and supports and regulates the immune system in both acute and chronic immunological dysfunctions. It is one of the best herbs for colds, influenza, and related infections of the ears, nose, and throat. Its powerful *tridoshic* balancing energy makes it very effective in the treatment of serious conditions like systemic *lupus erythematosus*, due to its affinity to the skin, blood, and joints.

A starchy water extract made from the solidified decoction of this herb is known as *gulwel sattva* or *giloy sattva*. This purified essence acts faster than the plain herb and can be used effectively during acute conditions, whereas the dried root has a slower and more sustained action. *Gulwel sattwa* is light, easily digestible, builds tissues, improves eyesight, and promotes intelligence and longevity.

Guduchi can be very effective for *pitta* related menstrual conditions, characterized by profuse menstruation, dysmenorrhea, vaginal irritation, and irritability, as well a yeast infections, especially when combined with the herbs *shatavari*, *vidari*, and *ashoka*. If yeast is an issue, then add herbs like *vidanga*, *shardunika,* licorice, or turmeric.

Guduchi is also referred to as *kaishore* and is the leading herb in the compound *kaishore guggulu*, which is useful for the treatment of *pitta* related conditions such as arthritis, gout, neuromuscular pain and inflammation, hypothyroidism, hyperthyroidism, skin diseases, *vata/pitta* menstrual complaints, and more. (See *Kaishore guggulu*.)

Guggul, Guggulu

Commiphora mukul; Burseaceae

Effect on Doshas: V- P+ (in excess) K-
Rasa: bitter, pungent, astringent, sweet Virya: heating Vipak: pungent
Preparations: See *Guggulu Preparations*.
Dosage: 1-6 g per day; pill or tablet, 250- 500 mg 2-3 times per day.

Parts used: purified resin.

Tissues: acts upon all tissues.

Systems: nervous, circulatory, digestive, musculoskeletal, respiratory, reproductive.

Properties: rejuvenative, nervine, antispasmodic, carminative, emmenagogue, stimulant, alterative, digestive, diaphoretic, diuretic, analgesic, expectorant, astringent, antiseptic, laxative, aphrodisiac.

Indications: arthritis, rheumatism, gout, nervous disorders, dyspepsia, GI tract diseases, obesity, high cholesterol, lumbago, repetitive motion injuries, heart and vascular conditions, neurasthenia, debility, diabetes, bronchitis, whooping cough, hemorrhoids, skin diseases, sores and ulcers, endometriosis, leucorrhea, cystitis, tumors, lymphatic congestion.

Precautions: high *pitta*, acute kidney infections (unless properly formulated), acute rashes.

Guggulu resin is an invaluable medicine in the Ayurvedic *pharmacopeia* because of its powerful cleansing and rejuvenating properties. It is often viewed as having similar qualities as myrrh, even though guggul is purified through a specialized herbal soaking procedure, making it gentler and easier to digest and eliminate from the system than other resinous herbal medicines.

It is often used as a natural binding agent in forming pills and it acts as a *yogavahi*, or catalytic agent, to enhance the properties of herbs that it is combined with and to direct their actions to specific tissues.

It is the primary herb in a class of guggulu compounds that are the treatment of choice for arthritic and inflammatory conditions and are also used for a wide variety of problems, including disorders of the muscle, joint, and bone tissues, as well as of the digestive, circulatory, urinary, and nervous systems. For instance, *kanchanar guggulu* is effective in reducing accumulations of *kapha* and *ama* in the fat and lymphatic tissue and is used to treat lymphadenopathy, tumors, cysts, and fibroids. Other compounds, such as *triphala guggulu*, are good for combating conditions like high cholesterol, abscesses, obesity, and diverticulosis, and *punarnavadi guggulu* for skin diseases, edema, and urinary disorders, amongst other complications.

Guggulu helps to kindle *agni* and improve the appetite, and does *mala shuddhi*, or cleansing of the waste products—urine, feces, and sweat. It disinfects and deobstructs the bowels, purifies bodily secretions, decongests thickened intestinal mucus and respiratory congestion caused by increased *kapha*, promotes absorption, and is curative in many chronic intestinal diseases.

Guggulu has a special affinity to the musculoskeletal and nervous systems. Depending on the herbs it is combined with, it helps to treat almost all forms of arthritis, as well as gout, osteoporosis, lumbago, fibromyalgia, neurological diseases, and generalized aches and pains.

It increases white blood cell count and purifies *rasa* and *rakta dhatus* (plasma/lymph and blood tissues), and is used to treat chronic respiratory disorders, urinary tract infections, skin diseases, and poor immunity.

Topically, it can be made into a paste with substances like lime juice and coconut oil to heal ulcers and hard-to-heal wounds. Used as a gargle, it cures gingivitis, chronic tonsillitis, and ulcers of the mouth and throat.

HARITAKI

Terminalia chebula; Combretacea

CHEBULIC MYROBALAN

Effect on Doshas: VPK=
Rasa: all except salty **Virya:** hot **Vipak:** sweet
Preparations: infusion, decoction, *gandarva haritaki* (haritaki roasted in castor oil), jam.
Dosage: 3-9 g per day.

Parts used: fruit.

Tissues: acts upon all tissues.

Systems: digestive, respiratory, excretory, nervous.

Properties: rejuvenative, digestive, astringent, laxative, nervine, expectorant, anthelmintic, antispasmodic.

Indications: cough, asthma, hoarseness of voice, flatus, abdominal distention, malabsorption, constipation, eye diseases, liver weakness, spleen diseases, jaundice, heart disease, skin diseases, nervous system disorders, edema, diarrhea, parasites, prolapsed organs, rheumatoid arthritis, high cholesterol, hemorrhage, skin ulcers, leucorrhea, spermatorrhea, obesity.

Precautions: high *pitta* (in excess), pregnancy, severe exhaustion, dehydration.

It is said that when the god Indra was drinking nectar in heaven, a drop fell to Earth and manifested as haritaki. Haritaki is regarded in Ayurvedic pharmacology as one of the best rejuvenative tonics for *vata dosha*. It strengthens the senses, nourishes the mind and nervous system, and promotes intelligence and longevity.

Haritaki is light and easy to digest, and contains five of the six tastes.

Its *prabhava* (special quality) is that it pacifies all three *doshas* and nourishes all bodily tissues, but it can provoke *pitta* when used in excess. Its hot quality stimulates *agni* and aids in the removal of blockages of the bodily channels caused by *ama* accumulation. Its astringency helps to tonify the GI tract, especially the colon, raise prolapsed organs, prevent and heal hemorrhoids, and prevent excessive bodily discharges in the case of urinary incontinence, leucorrhea, and spermatorrhea.

It is commonly used to increase the digestion and absorption of vital nutrients, burn toxins, dispel flatus, and promote regular bowel movements and healthy and well formed stool. It helps to cleanse and nourish *rasa dhatu* (plasma and lymphatic tissue), therefore enhancing the health and complexion of the top layer of the skin, which is its superior byproduct.

Haritaki is a fairly dynamic and versatile herb. For example, it can aid in weight loss by burning excess *kapha* when used with hot, pungent herbs like ginger, black pepper, or *pippali*, or to gain weight by promoting good absorption of nutrients if combined with warming carminatives like *ajwan*, ginger, nutmeg, cardamom, and tonic herbs like *ashwagandha*, *vidari*, or *bala*.

It is one of the three herbs that make up the traditional compound *triphala,* along with its partners *amalaki* and *bibhitaki*. *Triphala* can be used in much the same way as haritaki, but is more balanced and can be used by all body types and in most conditions where there is constipation or malabsorption. (See *Triphala*.)

When taken alone or in the *triphala* compound, it also helps to treat eye diseases and general weakness of vision. For this, it can also be taken either with honey, in the form of *triphala ghee*, as an eyewash, or alone with hot water.

The traditional Ayurvedic preparation known as *gandarva haritaki* (haritaki fried in castor oil) is quite effective for constipation due to increased *vata*, characterized by dry and hard stool, as well as in (*ama vata*) rheumatoid arthritis. This can be made at home by frying 4 parts of haritaki powder in 1 part castor oil in a cast iron skillet on a low heat until the herb is slightly browned. It can be taken at bedtime in 1/2 to 1 tsp. doses with hot water.

Agastya rasayana is another famous tonic containing haritaki. It is used to treat a wide variety of respiratory complaints and digestive disorders, including bronchitis, asthma, tuberculosis, allergies, sinusitis, coughs, and constipation. Unlike most *rasayanas*, which are given only after detoxification has taken place, *agasya rasayana* can be used even if there is *ama* present. It helps to bolster and strengthen the body's own healing response against even serious diseases.

HAWTHORNE BERRY

Crataegus oxycantha; Rosaceae

Effect on Doshas: V- PK+
Rasa: sour **Virya:** heating **Vipak:** sour, heavy
Preparations: decoction, infusion, jam, herbal wine.
Dosage: 1-12 g per day; tincture, 30 60 drops; solid extract, 1/4-1/2 tsp.

Parts used: fruit.

Tissues: plasma, blood, muscle.

Systems: circulatory, digestive.

Properties: carminative, stimulant, vasodilator, diuretic, tonic.

Indications: heart disorders, arteriosclerosis, dysrhythmia, hypertension, palpitations, angina, valvular insufficiency, blood clots, tumors, impacted wastes, debility, old age, gout.

Precautions: gastrointestinal ulcers, colitis.

Hawthorne berry is commonly used as a heart tonic, but its sour taste indicates that it possesses digestive qualities as well. It has warming and stimulating properties and is a mild coronary vasodilator, thereby increasing blood supply to the heart muscles. It is pacifying to *vata* and *kapha doshas* and increases *pitta* due to its heating action.

It can be used in the treatment of arteriosclerosis, hypertension, blood clots, arrhythmia, and extra systole. Its tonic action can help to stimulate heart function in deficient conditions, or depress it in conditions of excess. For lowering diastolic blood pressure, it combines well with equal parts *arjuna*, passionflower, and motherwort. One tsp. of this mixture steeped in a cup of hot water can be taken 3 times daily with raw honey. Even though hawthorne berry can increase *pitta*, it still can be used in a well balanced formula to support healthy heart function, providing that the person does not have both a *pitta* constitution and a *pitta* imbalance simultaneously, as in this case it could contribute to the *vikruti* or imbalance.

Hawthorne's effect on the heart is not only at the physical level. Its heart opening and warming qualities also help to bring unresolved emotions into the light of awareness and when combined with other herbs that have an affinity to the heart, it can have profound effects. A heart opening formula can be made by mixing it with equal parts *arjuna*, elecampane, and gotu kola.

It helps to pull uric acid from the tissues and has proven to be useful in the treatment of gout. As a digestive herb, it does *deepana*, or kindling of the digestive *agni*, *pachana*, or promoting digestion, and *bhedana*, or breaking down accumulated or impacted food masses and even tumors in the GI tract. In moderation, it can help to treat *manda agni* (slow digestion), caused by increased *kapha*, and is effective at trimming high cholesterol levels. It can be made into a wine with other digestive herbs for use before or after meals.

Hawthorne berry helps the body to utilize vitamin C and, being rich in bioflavonoids, is considered to possess antioxidant properties. Much like the *amalaki* fruit, it helps to strengthen, repair, and promote the growth of bodily tissues.

For treating disorders of the digestive system it combines well with cumin, fennel, peppermint, celery seed or *ajwan*, and ginger.

Other herbs to consider along with hawthorne for the heart include *arjuna*, broom, elecampane (*pushkaramula*), *punarnava*, passionflower, lily of the valley, mistletoe, motherwort, *tagara*, and foxglove.

JATAMANSI

Nardostachys jatamansi; Valerianaceae

INDIAN SPIKENARD

Effect on Doshas: VPK=
Rasa: bitter, sweet, slightly astringent **Virya:** cooling **Vipak:** sweet
Preparations: infusion, decoction (low simmer).
Dosage: 3-9 g per day.

Parts used: rhizome, roots.

Tissues: plasma, blood, muscle, nerve and marrow.

Systems: nervous, circulatory, urinary, digestive, respiratory.

Properties: nervine, relaxant, antispasmodic, vasodilator, anti-inflammatory, alterative, bitter tonic, diuretic, anticonvulsant.

Indications: anxiety, depression, spasms, convulsions, epilepsy, hypertension, hypotension, palpitations, arrhythmia, diminished appetite, motion sickness, jetlag, hepatitis, thrombophlebitis, skin eruptions, memory loss, hysteria, PMS, insomnia.

Jatamansi is a *tridoshic* rejuvenative for the nervous system that shares the calming quality of valerian, its close Western relative, without creating dullness of the body or mind. It has affinities to the mind, nerves, muscles, heart, liver, and GI tract. Its grounding effect on the mobile, erratic qualities of *vata* makes it useful in the treatment of anxiety, restlessness, spasms, tremors, convulsions, and even epilepsy.

It has a *sattwic* quality that helps to cool and pacify the mind, improve memory and concentration, and enhance awareness. It is useful for hyperactivity and the inability to focus, so it is especially helpful for children labeled ADD and ADHD. For this, it can be formulated with herbs like *ashwagandha*, *shankapushpi*, gingko, *brahmi*, and *vacha*.

When combined with equal parts *vacha* (calamus), it revitalizes the mind and nervous system and balances *vata* and *kapha*. Its calming and stabilizing action helps to improve the functional integrity of *prana vayu*, the vital breath, and *vyana vayu*, the aspect of *vata* present in the heart, whose role is to carry nutrients throughout the body via *rasa* and *rakta dhatu*. It helps to relax the heart muscles and is a mild vasodilator used in the treatment of hypertension and hypotension (especially when *vata* related), arrhythmia, and heart palpitations. In those cases, it combines well with *ashwagandha*.

Jatamansi's antispasmodic action helps to relieve premenstrual discomfort and generalized muscle and nervous tension. For menstrual disorders accompanied by cramping, bloating, or scanty menstruation, it can be combined with herbs like *musta* (nut grass), black cohosh, *shatavari*, *manjista*, and *vidari*. It has also proven useful in decreasing symptoms associated with menopause, such as mild to variable hot flashes, mood swings, insomnia, and generalized aches and pains.

Aside from being a calming and stress reducing herb, its bitter taste and cooling action make it useful for treating skin conditions like eczema, psoriasis, urticaria, hives, and other rashes. Due to the strong emotional component often associated with skin conditions, it works well to provide both blood cleansing as well as nervine properties.

Jatamansi is helpful in the treatment of hepatitis, for which it combines well with herbs like milk thistle and dandelion, as well as *kutki*, gentian, *guduchi*, *neem*, and *shankapushpi*.

When combined with equal parts dried ginger, it helps to promote appetite and relieve colic. Likewise, two 'OO' size capsules of this mixture can be taken before or during airplane flights or long bus rides to calm *vata* dosha and prevent jetlag.

For intestinal worms, it can be given with purgatives such as cascara, rhubarb, or *haritaki*.

Combined with a small amount of cinnamon and edible camphor, it can be used to support the treatment of bronchitis and other respiratory complaints. It has long been used in medicinal incense recipes to purify the atmosphere.

Jatamansi is commonly used in hair oils to promote hair health, along with herbs like *amalaki*, *brahmi*, and *bhringaraj*. *Jatamansi attar*, which is the essential oil in a sandalwood base, is a special anointing oil that is very useful for preventing *vata* imbalance when traveling and helps to induce a sound sleep for folks of all ages, including kids.

Just apply it to the temples and third eye, as needed.

Due to over harvesting, jatamansi is a threatened herb that is becoming increasingly difficult to find and to justify using. With the help of some ethically minded herb companies, efforts are being made to preserve and cultivate it. A good substitute for it is combining equal parts *tagara* and *shankapushpi*.

Kalmegh, Kalmegha

Andrographis paniculata; Acanthaceae
ANDROGRAPHIS

Effect on Doshas: **V+ (in excess) PK-**
Rasa: bitter **Virya:** cooling **Vipak:** pungent
Preparations: infusion.
Dosage: 1-6 g per day.

Parts used: whole plant.

Tissues: plasma, blood, fat.

Systems: digestive, circulatory.

Properties: alterative, antiviral, antipyretic, diuretic, stimulant, stomachic, bitter tonic, anthelmintic, febrifuge, cholagogue.

Indications: sluggish liver function, obesity, jaundice, dysentery, flatulence, abdominal distension, loss of appetite, colds, influenza, sinusitis, upper respiratory infections, dyspepsia, general debility, intermittent and remittent fever, malaria, convalescence after fever, neuralgia, parasites, ulcers, skin diseases, vitiligo, hemorrhoids.

Precautions: high *vata*, pregnancy, lactation.

Kalmegh is a powerful immunostimulant commonly used in the treatment of colds, influenza, and upper respiratory infections. Its antipyretic and antiviral properties also make it useful in cases of malaria, as well as any fever of an intermittent or remittent nature.

It helps to burn and eliminate *ama*, enhances liver function, stimulates bile flow, and is used to treat a wide variety of liver and spleen disorders, lymphatic congestion, as well as viral and bacterial infections. As a cholagogue, it can help to treat constipation caused by stagnant *pitta* in the liver and gallbladder, by stimulating bile flow. It has cleansing and rejuvenating effects on the blood and skin, which make it also useful for the treatment of vitiligo, eczema, and psoriasis.

Kalmegh helps to kindle *agni*, improves the appetite, and relieves flatulence, bloating, and irregular bowel movements caused by *ama*. It kills parasites and is also quite effective in the treatment of advanced dysentery. It is a good herb to decrease *kapha* in *meda dhatu* (fat tissue) and *mutra vaha srotas* (urinary system), and thus can help with edema and obesity, especially when combined with herbs like *punarnava*, *chitrak*, or dandelion leaf. It is a good substitute for the Ayurvedic herb *kutki*, a threatened Indian herb often used to scrape excess *kapha* from the system.

When used in excess, kalmegh may provoke the light, dry, and rough qualities of *vata*. Therefore, it is often used in formulation to balance its effect and enhance its action.

KAPI KACCHU

Mucuna pruriens; Fabaceae

ATMAGUPTA

Effect on Doshas: VP- K+
Rasa: sweet, bitter **Virya:** heating **Vipak:** sweet
Preparations: infusion, decoction, extract.
Dosage: 3-15 g per day.

Parts used: seeds.

Tissues: all tissues, most notably muscle, nerve, and reproductive.
Systems: reproductive, nervous, digestive.

Properties: aphrodisiac, antispasmodic, carminative, nervine.

Indications: general debility, depleted tissues, low libido, infertility, spermatorrhea, impotence, tics, tremors, spasms, Parkinson's disease, digestive discomfort, flatulence.

Precautions: high *ama* and profuse congestion.

Kapi kacchu is known in Ayurveda as one of the leading herbs for rejuvenating the reproductive system of both men and women. It rivals even the famous *ashwagandha* in its ability to enhance sexual stamina and vitality. It is not simply a sexual stimulant, but a nourishing tonic to the entire reproductive system.

For women's gynecological or reproductive conditions, it combines well with other versatile tonic herbs like *shatavari* or *vidari*; with musta, valerian, or cramp bark for menstrual cramping and discomfort, and with blood movers like *manjista*, motherwort, black cohosh, and saffron to promote normal menstrual flow.

To aid in male reproductive health, it is often combined with herbs like *ashwagandha*, *shilajit*, *shatavari*, and *vidari*.

It has an anabolic effect, thus improving the tone and strength of the muscle tissue and is specific for *mamsa gata-vata*, where *vata dosha* has increased and spread into the muscle tissue causing stiffness, fatigue, tics, tremors, spasms, and loss of strength and tone. It is often used along side tonic herbs like *ashwagandha*, *bala*, and *vidari* to calm *vata* and bring back tone and coordination.

It has a long history of use for *vata* related conditions of the nervous system, such as *kampavata* or Parkinson's disease and similar conditions that present with tremors and rigidity, but with no clear diagnosis. Recently this herb has been given a lot of attention, due to modern research showing that the seed contains L-dopa, an essential precursor to dopamine. Although it is questionable whether there is a known cure for this disease, this herb can aid tremendously in reducing the need for increasing strong medications and those who need them to respond better to treatment. It combines well with herbs that help to pacify the muscle and nerve tissues such as *brahmi*, gotu kola, valerian, *jatamansi*, and *ashwagandha*.

It also relieves gas and abdominal discomfort caused by excess *vata* and acts as a mild laxative due to its oily and spreading qualities. Here it can be prepared as a warm tea along with herbs like ginger, chamomile, fennel, *ajwan*, and *chitrak*.

Kutki

Picrorhiza kurroa; Scrophullariaceae

Effect on Doshas: V+ PK-
Rasa: bitter, pungent Virya: cooling Vipak: pungent
Preparations: infusion, decoction, medicated *ghee.*
Dosage: 1.5-3 g per day.

Parts used: root.

Tissues: plasma, blood, muscle.

System: circulatory, digestive, excretory, immune.

Properties: alterative, bitter tonic, antipyretic, antibacterial, anthelmintic, laxative, lithotriptic.

Indications: hepatitis, jaundice, fever, febrile debility, enlargement of the liver and spleen, herpes, shingles, acne, rashes, obesity, venereal sores, vitiligo, diabetes, cancer, lipoma, fibrocystic changes, high cholesterol, nausea, vomiting, obesity, parasites, colds, influenza.

Precautions: high *vata*, tissue deficiencies, variable or nervous digestion, diarrhea, hypoglycemia.

Kutki pacifies both *pitta* and *kapha*, and helps to rid the body of *ama*.

It is extremely effective for inflammatory problems, high fevers, and a variety of *pitta* related disorders rooted in the *rakta vaha srotas*—the channel of blood. It helps to purge excess *pitta* from the liver and gallbladder, and is indicated in hyperactive conditions of the liver and spleen. It is one of the main herbs for treating jaundice, all types of hepatitis, and for preventing cirrhotic changes.

Kutki helps to improve thyroid function and increase metabolism of proteins, cholesterol, and fats. It does *lechana*, or scraping of fat tissue, and is useful in cases of obesity, fibroids, fatty degenerative changes of the liver, high cholesterol and triglycerides, and hyperglycemia. For the management of obesity and related disorders, it combines well with other *kapha* reducing herbs like *chitrak* and *punarnava*. To dissolve or prevent gallstones, it can be mixed with herbs like dandelion, *manjista*, milk thistle, turmeric, and *chitrak*.

It rids the body of worms, but should be used with care, as it can lower libido by destroying sperm when used in excess or in high doses. It is one of the best herbs for treating high or chronic fevers, stubborn infections, and to support immune function. For lowering fevers, it can be mixed with such herbs as ginger, cinnamon, black pepper, or *tulsi*.

Kutki is a valuable remedy for herpes, genital herpes and sores, shingles, and venereal diseases like syphilis. It acts as a bitter tonic for *pitta* types of digestive complaints, especially when there is a difficulty digesting fatty food.

Due to over harvesting, kutki has become an increasingly endangered plant in India. For this reason, it is best to use substitutes for it whenever possible. Since it has a very similar action to both gentian and kalmegh (*andrographis paniculata)*, these can be used as good alternatives.

LICORICE

Glycerrhiza glabra; Leguminosae
YASHTI MADHU

Effect on Doshas: VP- K+ (in excess)
Rasa: sweet, bitter **Virya:** cooling **Vipak:** sweet
Preparations: infusion, decoction, milk decoction, medicated ghee
Dosage: 1-9 g per day; tincture, 30-60 drops.

Parts used: root.

Tissues: all tissues.

Systems: respiratory, digestive, reproductive, nervous.

Properties: demulcent, expectorant, emollient, tonic, laxative, emetic, anti-inflammatory, vulnerary, nourishing tonic.

Indications: coughs, colds, congestion, bronchitis, laryngitis, catarrhal conditions, sore throat, hyperacidity, urinary tract infections, fatigue, debility, adrenal exhaustion, painful urination, abdominal pain, peptic and skins ulcers.

Precautions: high *kapha*, chronic heart or kidney conditions, edema, hypertension (it can increase the water element around the heart), although small amounts of licorice may be safely used as a harmonizing herb in heart formulas. Be aware that many of the research studies on licorice have been done using the standardized extract on mice, which is <u>not</u> the whole herb in a human body.

Licorice is truly an invaluable medicine with a wide variety of uses in both Eastern and Western herbalism. It has cooling, demulcent, and expectorant properties, thereby helping to liquefy and expel phlegm and soothe dry coughs and inflamed bronchioles during upper respiratory tract infections. In cold, wet conditions, it combines well with warming herbs like osha root, ginger, or *pushkaramula* (elecampane). When combined with ginger alone, it makes a simple but remarkably effective home remedy for coughs, colds, congestion, and sinus congestion, as well as digestive complaints. It is a strengthening and revitalizing *rasayana* to the lungs that blends well with *pushkaramula* or *kantakari*.

Its soft, moistening, and cooling qualities also help to soothe inflammatory conditions of the GI tract, including gastritis, peptic ulcer, and ulcerative colitis, for which it is good combined with marshmallow root, comfrey root, and *shatavari*. Soaking a small amount of the root overnight to make a cold infusion to be taken in the morning with a little rice gruel can help to heal peptic ulcers.

Licorice can also be useful for constipation caused by an increased dry quality in the colon, and it is sometimes combined with other laxatives, including the traditional compound *triphala*, for this purpose.

It is a good adrenal tonic for those who have exhausted their energy stores from overworking, stressful lifestyles, or abusing stimulants like coffee, tea, or recreational drugs. For bolstering strength and energy, it combines nicely with other rejuvenative tonic herbs like *ashwagandha*, *bala*, or *shatavari*, and it has also proven useful relieving muscle or joint pain, as well as general fatigue.

Licorice can also aid in the treatment of *pitta* related disorders of the genitourinary tract like cystitis and vaginitis. For this, licorice tea or licorice medicated *ghee* is commonly used in *uttara basti* (douching) to cleanse and reduce inflammation and irritation. A simple douching preparation can be made by decocting 1 tsp. of the powdered root in 1 pint of water, straining it well, and douching once it is lukewarm. This can be repeated daily for short periods of time during an acute urinary or vaginal yeast infection and is a nice addition to a holistic and constitutional approach.

In large doses, licorice is an emetic and can induce vomiting. In Ayurvedic *vamana* therapy it is often used along with other emetic herbs including *vacha* (calamus), *madanphala* (emetic nut), and salt to expel phlegm and *ama* from the lungs and stomach. This is done only when the body has been properly prepared for such a radical cleansing, as during *Panchakarma*.

Licorice *ghee* can be used to protect and restore the bodily tissues. It works well when taken internally in doses from 1 tsp. to 1-2 Tblsp.

mixed into warm water or milk twice daily. It can also be applied to burns or skin ulcers and covered with sterile gauze (changed twice daily until ulcers are healed).

To heal corns on the feet, mix the powdered root with ground sesame seeds and a little mustard oil to make a paste. This can be applied to the hardened skin at bedtime and covered to soften and reduce growths.

When a small amount of licorice is added to a formula it acts to harmonize the other herbs and enhance the overall action of the formula. It is often used to mask strong or nasty tasting herbs and to counter herbs that have rough and irritating qualities.

The sweet taste of licorice is thought to awaken positive cellular memory and bring satisfaction and contentment to the mind. When combined with herbs that have an affinity to the mind and nervous system it helps to invoke a calming energy.

A stick of licorice is tasty to chew on and can be used to make a natural toothbrush to clean the teeth. It also helps to enhance the voice and is nice when combined with cardamom, ginger, and powdered sugar. This is a good herb to keep around the kitchen since kids generally love it with a little honey.

Lobelia

Lobelia inflata; Lobeliaceae

Effect on Doshas: VP+ K-
Rasa: pungent, astringent **Virya:** heating **Vipak:** pungent
Preparations: infusion, tincture.
Dosage: 3-12 g per day; tincture, 10 to 30 drops.

Parts used: aerial parts.

Tissues: plasma, nervous.

Systems: lymphatic, respiratory, nervous.

Properties: antispasmodic, diaphoretic, emetic, expectorant, respiratory stimulant (in small doses), relaxant (in large doses), nervine.

Indications: asthma, bronchitis, spasmodic coughs, spasms, neuralgia, poisoning, nervous tension.

Precautions: skilled supervision is necessary when using this herbs as an emetic.

For centuries, lobelia has been a well known but rather controversial herb in Western herbalism, due to its use as an emetic. Yet when used skillfully, considering proper energetic and constitutional guidelines, it can be a valuable and safe medicine. It is a powerful *kapha* pacifying herb with an affinity to the respiratory tract and the stomach, which are the main sites of *kapha*.

It helps to clear obstructions and increase the flow of the vital *prana*. It is an effective expectorant and antispasmodic used in the treatment of respiratory complaints, and has a depressant action on the central and autonomic nervous system. It acts as a stimulant in smaller doses, and in moderate to larger doses it has a relaxant action.

Because it has both stimulant and relaxant properties, one of its most well known uses is for the treatment of asthma and bronchial congestion. It stimulates the secretion and expectoration of phlegm, while also helping to relax the muscles of the respiratory tract, and has long been used by Western herbalists as a cleansing emetic, although with some debate as to its safety. When administered in large doses of 1-2 tsp. or more of the tincture, it does induce vomiting, and can therefore purge phlegm from the lungs while helping to relax the bronchioles. It has been proven to stop an asthma attack and in some cases has been noted to prevent future attacks.

It is worth noticing that this approach for asthma may not be safe and effective for everyone, so it must always be administered from a constitutional perspective, considering what treatment is best suited to the individual constitution (*prakruti*) while keeping the present state of the *doshas* (*vikruti*) in mind.

In the traditional Ayurvedic cleansing program known as *Panchakarma*, one of the five main cleansing measures is *vamana chikitsa* (or emetic therapy), which is administered only when indicated, on a case by case basis, and only after the body has been properly prepared for this procedure. The unique aspect of employing *vamana chikitsa* during *Panchakarma* is that excess *kapha* and *ama* are first coaxed out of the deep tissues and then encouraged to move toward the GI tract. After this, vomiting not only dispels *ama* that is already present in the stomach, but also that which will continue to arrive there throughout the cleansing process, as it sets in motion the flow of *kapha* and *ama* out of the body (like a siphon), making it easier for the body to efficiently deal with the *ama* still circulating in all the systems.

Using lobelia as an emetic is indicated mainly for *kapha* related respiratory complaints characterized by excess phlegm accumulated in the lungs and stomach. Drinking a stimulating cup of peppermint, ginger, and cinnamon tea to support the process can precede emetic therapy using lobelia. This approach should only be done with the guidance of a practitioner skilled in *Panchakarma* therapies.

If asthma is caused by increased *vata*, characterized by wheezing, tightness in the chest and scanty mucus, vomiting therapy is not advised, but smaller doses of lobelia may still be used in a formulation as a supportive and catalyzing herb to help relax and open the airways. One of my favorite asthma formulas can be prepared by steeping 3 heaping Tbsp. mullein (cut herb), 1 Tbsp. *tulsi (cut herb)*, and 1/2 to 1 tsp. licorice (powder) in 1 quart of hot water for 30 minutes, straining, and adding 30 drops of lobelia tincture and 1-2 tsp. raw honey. Drink 1 cup 3-4 times daily, as needed.

Inhalation of the smoke of this herb can also help to open the bronchioles during the first onset of an asthma attack. Smoking a little lobelia is also thought to diminish the craving for nicotine.

Manjista

Rubia cordifolia-radix; Rubiaceae
INDIAN MADDER

Effect on Doshas: V+ PK-
Rasa: bitter, sweet, astringent **Virya:** cooling **Vipak:** pungent
Preparations: infusion, decoction, medicated oil and *ghee*, paste.
Dosage: 3-9 g per day.

Parts used: roots.

Tissues: plasma, blood, muscle, bone, reproductive.

Systems: circulatory, female reproductive, urinary, bone.

Properties: alterative, hemostatic, emmenagogue, diuretic, anti-inflammatory, lithotriptic, antitumor, vulnerary.

Indications: skin disorders, itching, acne, amenorrhea, dysmenorrhea, menorrhagia, endometriosis, menopause, herpes, bleeding disorders, broken bones, kidney or gallstones, hepatitis, jaundice, dysentery, cancer, heart disease, paralysis, dropsy, rickets, chronic wounds, scabies, fungal infections, athlete's foot, ulcers.

Precautions: high *vata*.

Manjista is a rich red colored root with a special affinity to the blood, as well as many other *pitta* specific regions of the body. It cleanses and improves liver and spleen functions and is unsurpassed for dealing with obstinate skin disorders caused by toxic blood, including eczema, psoriasis, dermatitis, herpes, acne, boils, rosacea, hives, athlete's foot, and scabies. Here it combines well with other blood cleansing herbs like *neem* and turmeric. It also pacifies *kapha*, which often plays a secondary role in inflammatory skin conditions, especially swollen, weeping types of eczema or psoriasis.

It cools and moves blood and is useful for *pitta* and *kapha* related gynecological problems. It has a dual action in that it calms menstrual pain, inflammation, and irritation, and checks profuse menstrual bleeding associated with excess *pitta*, while restoring normal flow in the case of uterine congestion from accumulated *kapha*.

Manjista also speeds up the healing of wounds and ulcers. As a hemostatic, it stops bleeding in both the GI and urinary tracts. For knitting broken bones, it combines well with *arjuna* or comfrey leaves.

Its *bhedana* (breaking) action helps to remove benign and malignant tumors, dissolve kidney and gallstones, and clear liver and kidney obstructions. Lastly, it helps with mental irritability and is good along side other anti-*pitta* herbs that have a stronger affinity to the mind and nervous system, such as skullcap, *shankapushpi*, or gotu kola to enhance its effect.

MARSHMALLOW

Althea officinalis; Malvaceae

Effect on Doshas: VP- K+
Rasa: sweet **Virya: cooling** **Vipak: sweet**
Preparations: decoction, infusion, milk decoction, paste.
Dosage: 3-15 g per day.

Parts used: primarily the roots.

Tissues: reproductive, plasma, blood, marrow and nerve.

Systems: respiratory, urinary, nervous, digestive, reproductive.

Properties: nutritive tonic, demulcent, expectorant, emollient, vulnerary, diuretic, laxative.

Indications: dry cough, whooping cough, sore throat, laryngitis, respiratory tract infection, inflammatory conditions of the kidneys and bladder, gastritis, ulcers, infections, skin eruptions, constipation, hyperacidity, diarrhea, cuts and wounds, tissue wasting, malnutrition, general debility.

Precautions: low *agni* (digestive fire), high *kapha* or *ama* conditions.

Marshmallow is highly mucilaginous and soothing to inflamed mucous membranes of the GI and urinary tract. It is a sweet, heavy, and nutritive tonic somewhat similar to its Indian relative *bala* (*Sida cordifolia*).

It is a pacifying and rejuvenating herb to *vata* and *pitta doshas*, and is helpful in disorders of the GI tract including gastritis, peptic ulcer, diarrhea, constipation, and ulcerative colitis, as it helps to absorb the hot, sharp, liquid, and spreading qualities of *pitta dosha*, while soothing and healing any damaged tissue. For this, it combines well with herbs like licorice, arrowroot, *shatavari*, or *guduchi*. I often use marshmallow as a substitute for licorice in cases where licorice may be contraindicated.

It can also be applied externally as a warm poultice to promote healing to minor cuts, wounds, hard-to-heal ulcers, and bedsores. It relieves discomfort during the elimination of kidney stones when used along with other diuretic and lithotriptic herbs.

Its moistening quality is good for treating constipation when caused by dryness in the colon, and it can be mixed with psyllium seed to enhance its effect.

As a tonic to *vata,* take it first thing in the morning on an empty stomach as a milk decoction, along with a pinch of ginger, cardamom, and saffron.

To tonify the lungs, it combines well with herbs like mullein, licorice, comfrey root, and elecampane, or in a milk decoction with turmeric. It is effective for soothing coughs and sore throat, and is a nice remedy for dry or whooping cough in children. To liquefy bronchial congestion, it can be mixed with expectorating herbs like ginger, osha, pippali, yerba santa, or elecampane (*pushkarmula*).

Meadow sweet

Filipendula ulmaria; Rosaceae

Effect on Doshas: V+ PK-
Rasa: bitter, astringent Virya: cooling Vipak: pungent
Preparations: infusion.
Dosage: 3-18 g per day; tincture, 30-60 drops.

Parts used: aerial portions.

Tissues: plasma, blood, muscle, fat.

Systems: digestive.

Properties: anti-rheumatic, anti-inflammatory, analgesic, digestive, antacid, carminative, antiemetic, astringent.

Indications: hyperacidity, peptic ulcers, gastritis, heartburn, nausea, food poisoning, arthritis, rheumatism, gout, muscle pain, fever, headaches.

Precautions: high *vata*.

Meadowsweet is a soothing herb for the digestive tract, especially for *pitta* disorders such as hyperacidity, gastritis, peptic ulcers, and nausea. Its mild astringency helps to reduce the hot, liquid, and sharp qualities of *pitta* in the stomach and small intestine, making it useful in treating diarrhea safely, even for children. A simple tea for *pitta* types of digestive problems can be made by steeping 1-2 tsp. of the cut leaf in 1 cup of hot water for 10 minutes and drinking after or between meals. It can also be combined with herbs like chamomile, lemon balm, and licorice.

Due to its bitter and astringent tastes and cold energy, it will suppress *agni* over time, so it is better to use it for short periods or with other herbs to balance its effects.

Meadowsweet can be considered the mother of aspirin, since salicylic acid was first isolated from this herb in 1838. It is safer than aspirin because the whole herb contains tannins and mucilage that buffer the irritating effects of salicylates, which can cause gastric irritation or bleeding when isolated from the herb. It is an effective pain reliever for sore joints, muscles, inflammatory arthritic conditions, and gout, and is also a useful remedy for headaches, fevers, colds, and the flu.

Milk Thistle

Silybum marianum; Asteraceae

Effect on Doshas: V+ PK-
Rasa: bitter and sweet Virya: cooling Vipak: pungent
Preparations: infusion, tincture.
Dosage: 1-9 g per day; tincture, 30-90 drops.

Parts used: seeds, aerial portions.

Tissues: plasma, blood, fat.

Systems: plasma, blood.

Properties: hepato-protective, cholagogue, alterative, anti-inflammatory, bitter tonic, demulcent, galactagogue, anti-toxic.

Indications: hepatitis, drug and alcohol poisoning, cirrhosis, hemorrhoids, portal hypertension, hydrocele, chronic urethritis, enlarged prostate, enlargement of the liver and spleen, varicose veins, alcoholism, Epstein-Barr virus, chronic fatigue, cytomegalovirus, Crohn's disease.

Precautions: high *vata*.

Milk thistle is clearly one of the best liver stimulating and protecting herbs in Western herbalism. From an Ayurvedic perspective, it is a great herb for kindling the *agni* principle present in the liver. The liver plays a major role in converting the five elements of food into biologically available forms of nourishment for the whole body through what is known as *bhuta agni*, or the fire component of the five elements. Liver enzymes are a main component of *bhuta agni*.

Milk thistle is good for *sama pitta* conditions, helping to clear excess heat and toxins from the liver and blood. It protects the liver from exposure to toxic chemicals, drugs and alcohol, and also from accumulated *ama* resulting from a poor diet and lifestyle. It is commonly used in Europe to prevent hangovers due to excess alcohol consumption. This little remedy has been known to give their Olympic skiers the edge over other countries after a night of partying and drinking.

It does *lechana* (scraping of fat) and is useful for fatty degenerative changes in the liver and treating gallbladder complaints. It also helps to clear pelvic congestion and can be combined well with herbs like kalmegh, *kutki*, or *neem* to relieve portal hypertension, which can lead to varicosities.

It is similar in action to the Ayurvedic herb *kutki*, which is "at risk" due to over harvesting in India. It is extremely useful in the treatment of mononucleosis, hepatitis, necrosis, and cirrhosis. One of the active principles in milk thistle is silymarin, which stimulates the regeneration of liver cells though protein synthesis. It is also used for enlargement of the liver and spleen. Some modern research is being done that indicates the possibility that milk thistle may inhibit the growth of breast, prostate, and cervical cancer cells.

Motherwort

Leonurus cardiaca; Labiatae

LION'S TAIL, THROW-WORT

Effect on Doshas: V+ PK-
Rasa: bitter, pungent **Virya:** cooling **Vipak:** pungent
Preparations: infusion, decoction, tincture.
Dosage: 1-9 g per day; tincture, 30- 60 drops.

Parts used: leaves.

Tissues: plasma, blood, muscle, nerve and marrow, reproductive.

Systems: circulatory, reproductive, nervous, urinary, digestive.

Properties: emmenagogue, cardiac tonic, digestive, nervine, antispasmodic, diuretic.

Indications: suppressed or delayed menstruation, heart disorders, arteriosclerosis, nervous tension, insomnia, convulsions, tachycardia, hysteria.

Precautions: avoid during pregnancy or profuse menstrual bleeding.

Motherwort's Latin botanical name is *Leonurus cardiaca*, which means "lion hearted," due to its calming and regulating effect on the heart. It is a mild vasodilator and is also useful in the treatment of cardiac edema, tachycardia, arteriosclerosis, blood clots, angina, and palpitations. I consider it to be a fairly *tridoshic* herb, but due to its cooling energy, it may increase *vata* in high doses, if taken over an extended period of time. For the heart, motherwort can be combined along with other herbs like elecampane, hawthorne berries, cardamom, and *arjuna*.

Motherwort is also a female supporting herb with emmenagogue properties that can be used to treat suppressed or irregular menses, painful uterine cramping with scanty menstrual flow, and water retention. Suppressed or delayed menses is often due to the erratic nature of *vata*, so a nice formula can be made by combining it with equal parts angelica and cramp bark along with 1/2 part ginger.

When taken right after pregnancy, it relaxes the uterus and helps it to return to normal tone. For this, it combines well with herbs like *ashoka* and red raspberry.

Women experiencing menopause may find it helpful for diminishing hot flashes and mood swings. Here, it is best combined with herbs like *shatavari* and *vidari*. Due to its emmenagogue properties, motherwort should not be used if there is heavy menstrual flow or during pregnancy, as it may cause uterine contractions.

Its nervine properties help to treat mental and emotional disturbances, convulsions, and occasional insomnia. For this, it combines well with herbs such as avena, valerian, skullcap, *ashwagandha*, and *jatamansi*.

MUSTA

Cyperus rotundus; Cyperaceae
NUTGRASS

Effect on Doshas: V+ (in excess) PK-
Rasa: pungent, bitter, astringent **Virya:** cooling **Vipak:** pungent
Preparations: decoction, infusion, oil.
Dosage: 1-9 g per day.

Parts used: rhizome.

Tissues: plasma, blood, muscle, marrow and nerve.

Systems: digestive, respiratory, nervous, circulatory, female reproductive.

Properties: nervine, antispasmodic, digestive, stimulant, carminative, astringent, alterative, analgesic, emmenagogue, anthelmintic.

Indications: menstrual disorders, PMS, dysmenorrhea, menopause, digestive disorders, malabsorption, indigestion, spasms, uterine cramping, diarrhea, sluggish liver function, headaches, candida, dysentery, colic, parasites, ulcers, gastritis, cholera.

Precautions: high *vata*, constipation.

Musta is a very useful digestive tonic for *pitta* individuals or disorders, as it helps to stimulate the appetite and digestion while clearing excess heat and *ama* from the small intestine. As such, it is an extremely effective herb for dealing with the root causes of candida and bacterial infections of the GI tract.

It is used for the treatment of fever, chronic diarrhea, dysentery, gastritis, cholera, nausea, vomiting, and intestinal parasites. A simple tea can be had at room temperature during the hot season to relieve summer heat. It makes a good beverage tea for *pitta* types while observing a 1 to 2 day juice fast or mono diet to promote detoxification. It is also diaphoretic and used to treat recurrent or relapsing fever and to appease thirst.

Musta is one of the best aids for female disorders. It helps to relieve cramping and fluid retention, move blood, and regulate the menstrual cycle. It works particularly well to ease emotional problems associated with PMS, and for this it combines well with equal parts skullcap.

For *pitta* types of female reproductive issues, it combines well with gotu kola and *shatavari*. If there is a tendency toward heavy bleeding, it can be combined with *ashoka* or raspberry leaf. For irregular or absent periods, it mixes well with *ashwagandha, shatavari,* angelica (*tang kuei*), wild yam, or *vidari*.

A nice female reproductive tonic is 5 parts *shatavari*, 4 parts *vidari* (or wild yam), 3 parts musta and angelica, and 2 parts ginger. One ounce of this mixture can be simmered in 1 quart of water for 20 minutes and taken in doses of 1 cup 3-4 times a day.

Taken with powdered ginger and raw honey, it helps to increase the appetite and digestion. It is also a good herb for relieving headaches, including migraines due to increased *pitta,* and combines well with herbs like feverfew, gotu kola, *jatamansi*, and all types of mint.

Musta is an affective pain reliever and can be used to treat low back pain and generalized stiffness and cramping. It makes a good substitute for valerian for such conditions, especially for individuals with *pitta* imbalances that might find valerian too heating and even stimulating. Otherwise, it combines well with *ashwagandha* and *tagara* (or valerian).

Myrrh

Commiphora myrrha; Burseraceae

BOLA

Effect on Doshas: VK- P+
Rasa: bitter, astringent, pungent **Virya:** heating **Vipak:** pungent
Preparations: infusion, powder, tincture, paste, pill, liniment.
Dosage: 1.5-12 g per day; tincture, 5-20 drops.

Parts used: gum resin.

Tissues: acts on all bodily tissues.

Systems: circulatory, reproductive, nervous, respiratory, lymphatic.

Properties: emmenagogue, alterative, tonic, expectorant, antispasmodic, rejuvenative, antiseptic, analgesic, astringent.

Indications: dysmenorrhea, amenorrhea, menopause, colds, cough, asthma, influenza, abscesses, infections, arthritis, rheumatism, bronchitis, sinusitis, gum disease, stomatitis, pyorrhea, pharyngitis, laryngitis, traumatic injuries, anemia, low immunity and vitality, poor circulation, uterine tumors.

Precautions: high *pitta* conditions, kidney disorders.

For thousands of years myrrh has been regarded in both Eastern and Western herbal traditions as both a rejuvenating and detoxifying substance. It is pacifying to *vata* and *kapha*, but may increase *pitta* if used in excess.

It has similar properties to *guggulu* (*commiphora mukul*), which is one of the most important *rasayanas* in Ayurvedic medicine. They both have affinities to the joints, blood, muscles, bones, nerves, and female reproductive system. It can be used to treat arthritic and rheumatic complaints, as well as circulatory disorders. It cleanses stagnant blood from the uterus and has a strong action on the nervous system.

Myrrh helps to burn *ama* from the body and promotes the formation of healthy tissue. It is well known for its anti microbial and antiseptic properties, making it useful in treating gingivitis, canker sores, tooth abscesses, sore throat, and a wide variety of infections. It stimulates phagocytosis and the prompt response of white blood cell to infection, making it supportive to the immune system's first line of defense. It is far more effective for colds, influenza, upper respiratory tract and sinus infections than antibiotics without the depleting effects on the intestinal tract and immune system.

Due to its tonic and rejuvenating properties, it increases *agni* without disturbing the balance of intestinal flora when used for extended periods of time. In acute situations, it combines well with stronger bitter herbs like goldenseal or echinacea to both enhance and balance their effect.

The powder can be made into a paste and applied topically to treat wounds, boils, and sores, and the diluted tincture can be used as an antiseptic mouthwash for disorders of the mouth, gums, and throat.

Myrrh is subtle and penetrating. It reaches deep into the body and can be considered a *yogavahi* (catalytic agent) that helps to potentiate and direct the energy of the herbs it is combined with. When burned along with frankincense, it purifies the atmosphere, the mind, and the subtle body.

Unlike myrrh, *guggulu* is put through a purification processes that makes it easier to absorb and eliminate from the body than myrrh in its raw form, which is thought to irritate the kidneys when used for extended periods of time.

Neem

Azadiracta indica; Meliaceae

Effect on Doshas: V+ PK-
Rasa: bitter Virya: cooling Vipak: pungent
Preparations: infusion, decoction, medicated *ghee* and oil, paste.
Dosage: 0.5-5 g per day.

Parts used: bark, leaves, fresh twigs.

Tissues: plasma, blood, fat.

Systems: digestive, circulatory, respiratory, urinary.

Properties: alterative, bitter tonic, antipyretic, anthelmintic, antiseptic, antiviral, anti-inflammatory.

Indications: skin diseases (eczema, psoriasis, skin cancer, urticaria, ring worm, etc.), liver disorders, parasites, hemorrhoids, fever, malaria, coughs, excess thirst (due to *pitta*), diabetes, tumors, cancer, obesity, high cholesterol, arthritis, jaundice, rheumatism, vomiting.

Precautions: high *vata*, cold and/or dry conditions, constipation, tissue deficiency, low libido.

Neem has a powerful cleansing action upon the liver, spleen, blood, and lymphatic system and is pacifying to *pitta* and *kapha*. It is effective in treating skin conditions such as urticaria, eczema, psoriasis, and other obstinate skin diseases. Washing with a strong infusion of the leaves, which are highly antiseptic and astringent, helps to promote the healing of wounds, infections, fungal infections, and foul or gangrenous ulcers. Because of its cleansing, purifying, and antibacterial properties, some companies have developed effective neem products such as soaps, shampoos, mouthwashes, tooth powders, creams and salves. A good sign that these products are high quality is that neem's bitterness is not masked by flavoring or fragrances.

It has a *pitta* reducing action upon the GI tract and is useful for hyperacidity and inflammatory bowel disorders, including Crohn's disease, ulcers, and colitis. It rids the body of all kinds of intestinal worms, as well as other parasites like ringworm, lice, and scabies. For skin parasites, it is good in a cream, oil, salve, or shampoo for local application. Care should be taken when using neem, because it can deplete the sperm when taken internally for prolonged periods.

Neem's antipyretic properties are effective in the treatment of chronic or intermittent fevers, for which it combines well with herbs like *tulsi*, coriander, ginger, and clove. As a preventative for malaria and parasites, neem can be taken daily in small doses while traveling in places where those can be a problem, such as India, South America, or Africa.

Its alterative and astringent actions help to reduce *kapha* and *ama*. When combined with herbs like *shardunika*, turmeric, or barberry, it is often used to regulate blood sugar levels, and is an important part of treatment in type 2 diabetes.

Neem works well to reduce swelling, discomfort, and bleeding associated with *pitta* types of hemorrhoids. In this case, it combines well with such herbs as *guduchi*, *manjista*, or barberry. Neem oil can be applied to the anal area in a coconut oil base to provide added relief.

The fresh or powdered leaves can be mixed with boiling water and a little raw honey to form a paste that can be applied to glandular swellings and boils. The medicated oil is a strong disinfectant for topical use and can also help to reduce joint and muscle pain and inflammation due to arthritis.

A strong, stinky smelling sap that is extracted from the fruit is used topically for obstinate skin diseases and to relieve itching. It is often mixed with turmeric for this purpose, although, in my experience, this pure extract is too strong to apply directly to rashes like eczema or psoriasis and should be diluted in a gentler base oil.

Nettle

Urtica urens; Urticaceae

Effect on Doshas: V+ PK-
Rasa: bitter, astringent, sweet Virya: cooling Vipak: pungent
Preparations: infusion, tincture, freeze dried herb.
Dosage: 6-30 g per day.

Parts used: aerial parts.

Tissues: plasma, blood, bone, nerve and marrow.

Systems: digestive, nervous, respiratory, urinary.

Properties: digestive bitter, diuretic, alterative, astringent, anti-inflammatory, homeostatic, tonic.

Indications: skin diseases, gout, bleeding disorders, arthritis, allergies, hay fever, uterine bleeding, eczema, psoriasis, asthma, nervous tension, hemorrhoids, digestive complaints, hair fall, liver conditions, urinary complaints, edema, obesity, fatigue caused by high *ama*.

Nettle is a nutrient rich herb that may be as beneficial as many of the more costly green food supplements found on the market nowadays. Its bitter and slightly astringent tastes help to reduce excess *kapha* and can be used to treat edema, respiratory congestion, and mucus accumulation in the stomach or colon. It also stimulates the secretion and removal of uric acid from the system and is extremely useful for treating gout and arthritic and rheumatic conditions.

It works quite well for *pitta* related skin conditions such as eczema and psoriasis, especially to calm itching brought on by stress, anxiety, and worry. Its mild astringency also helps to treat bleeding disorders such as nosebleeds, rectal spotting, bleeding hemorrhoids, and uterine bleeding, all of which may be symptoms of an increase of *pitta* in the general circulation.

Nettle helps to remove *ama* caused by poorly digested food, as well as from exposure to substances such as mold, dust, pollens, and chemicals, which can eventually contribute to environmental or food related allergies. For treating hay fever, asthma, and allergies in general, it can be combined with equal parts turmeric and *amalaki*.

Drinking the tea of fresh leaves in the springtime is a gentle and effective way to renew the system by helping to cleanse excess *kapha* and *ama* accumulated during the cold, damp winter months.

Nettle is a good blood and bone building tonic rich in iron, calcium, potassium, zinc, magnesium, and silica, as well as a variety of other vitamins and minerals. From an Ayurvedic perspective, it doesn't possess all of the qualities of a rejuvenating herb, and if used in excess it may increase *vata* and weaken the digestive fire over time, due to its cooling energy and astringent and bitter tastes. In my experience, it combines well with nourishing and rejuvenating tonic herbs to balance its effects, such as *amalaki, shatavari, vidari*, or wild yam.

For cleansing the liver, blood, and skin, it can be mixed with burdock and *neem*. With equal parts dandelion or coriander, it is extremely cleansing to the kidneys and urinary tract. To nourish and strengthen the kidneys and adrenals, it combines well with *gokshura,* gotu kola *(brahmi)* or licorice.

For indigestion caused by overindulgence of rich, fried, and heavy food, nettle can be mixed with other digestives herbs like ginger, chamomile, meadowsweet, or peppermint.

Nirgundi

Vitex negundo; Verbenaceae

Effect on Doshas: V- P+ (in excess) K-
Rasa: bitter, astringent, pungent Virya: heating (leaves), cooling (fruit, flowers, seeds) Vipak: pungent
Preparations: infusion, decoction, medicated oil.
Dosage: 3-9 g per day.

Parts used: root, flowers, leaf, fruit.

Tissues: plasma, blood, muscle, nerve and marrow, reproductive.

Systems: circulatory, digestive.

Properties: analgesic, anthelmintic, alterative, anti-inflammatory, bitter tonic, febrifuge, expectorant, nervine, emmenagogue, astringent, antiseptic, demulcent

Indications: rheumatoid arthritis, muscle pain, sprains, headaches, worms, wounds, ulcers, venereal diseases, fever, insect bites, cramps, spasms, obstructions, hemorrhoids.

Nirgundi leaves have a warming action. They act as a circulatory stimulant and are commonly used to relieve pain and inflammation of the muscles and joints due to *ama-vata* (rheumatoid arthritis), osteoarthritis, and sprains, as well as generalized aches and pains.

A decoction of nirgundi tea can also be used for *nadi swedana*, a localized steam therapy for such conditions. Here the medicated steam can be applied directly to specific areas of the body while massaging medicated oils such as *dashamoola* or *mahanarayan* oil to the site. The tea can also be added to a warm bath to achieve similar results, if needed.

Nirgundi essential oil is convenient for infusing the water in a steam cabinet. If the essential oil cannot be obtained, simply apply nirgundi oil locally to sore areas before entering the cabinet or bathtub.

The oil of the fresh leaves is useful to reduce glandular swellings and promote healing of wounds and necrotic tissues.

The leaves are also used internally for the treatment of rheumatism and can be mixed with other anti-inflammatory herbs such as garlic, *guggulu*, boswellia, turmeric, ginger, and *ajwan*.

When combined with equal parts *pippali*, *tulsi*, and ginger, it helps to burn *ama* from the *rasa dhatu*, thus relieving fever, sinus inflammation and congestion, and mental fatigue.

A warm poultice of the fresh or dried leaves can also be applied for relieving muscle, joint and neurological pain, and on the forehead and temples to relieve headaches.

The root bark is prepared as a tincture and also used in its powdered form for rheumatism, urinary disorders, hemorrhoids, dysentery, dyspepsia, colic, and worms.

The fruit and flowers are used in cases of *pitta* related diarrhea, cholera, fever, and liver diseases. The flowers are used also as a cardiac tonic and to stop bleeding in the GI tract.

NUTMEG

Myristica fragrans; Myristicaceae

JATIPHALA

Effect on Doshas: V- P+ K-
Rasa: pungent **Virya: heating** **Vipak: pungent**
Preparations: infusion, essential oil, medicated milk (not boiled).
Dosage: 0.5-6 g per day.

Parts used: fruit (seeds).

Tissues: plasma, muscle, marrow and nerve, reproductive.

Systems: digestive, nervous, reproductive.

Properties: astringent, analgesic, carminative, sedative, stimulant, nervine, aphrodisiac.

Indications: intestinal gas, abdominal pain, headaches, poor absorption, bloating, diarrhea, dysentery, nervous disorders, insomnia, impotence, urinary incontinence, premature ejaculation, uterine disorders.

Precautions: high *pitta*, pregnancy.

Nutmeg is a common kitchen spice and a valuable Ayurvedic medicine. It is often used as a sedative, digestive stimulant, and carminative to calm and correct *vata* in the colon and nervous system. It is quite useful to treat flatulence, bloating, abdominal pain, and malabsorption. For this, 1/2 tsp. of a mixture of equal parts nutmeg, dried ginger, and *ajwan* can be taken before meals.

Its astringent properties make it particularly useful for diarrhea. A simple and effective recipe for this, which can be taken twice a day, is made by steaming and mashing 2 apples and adding in 1/2 tsp. nutmeg powder and 1 tsp. *ghee*. For treating diarrhea caused by summer heat, it can be taken with buttermilk.

Nutmeg is also helpful for treating spasmodic coughs, nervous tension, and muscle spasms. For insomnia caused by increased *vata dosha*, a cup of warm milk with a pinch or two of nutmeg can be taken before bed to calm and relax body and mind. However, it has a *tamasic* quality and is dulling to the mind when taken regularly in moderate to large doses.

A drop of nutmeg essential oil applied to the temples is beneficial for relieving headaches, especially those associated with nervous tension, anxiety, restlessness, or constipation. The essential oil can also be applied to specific *marma* points, combined in liniments, and infused in an herbal steam bath to ease muscular and joint pain.

It can help to pacify excess *vata* in the male reproductive tissue, thereby improving the tone of the male sexual organs, and correcting premature ejaculation. Here it can be taken with *ashwagandha*. It is also used to increase fertility and lessen menstrual pains in women. When taken after childbirth, it helps to normalize *apana vayu*, the downward moving aspect of *vata*. Its astringent properties also make it an effective remedy for urinary incontinence due to high *vata* and *kapha*.

There are many traditional formulas containing nutmeg, including *jatiphaladi gutika* and *jatiphaladi churnam*, which have *vata anuloman* (carminative) properties and are used to correct *vata* related digestive complaints, dysentery, spasmodic cough, asthma, and neuralgia.

Osha Root

Ligustacum porteri; Umbelliferae

Effect on Doshas: V- P+ K-
Rasa: pungent, bitter Virya: heating Vipak: pungent
Preparations: infusion, decoction, extract, cough syrup.
Dosage: 3 to 9 g per day; tincture, 20-60 drops.

Parts used: root

Tissues: plasma, blood, muscle, fat.

Systems: respiratory, digestive, immune.

Properties: expectorant, digestive, antimicrobial, antibiotic, diaphoretic.

Indications: colds, cough, sore throat, influenza, respiratory congestion, bronchitis, fever, infections, poor appetite.

Precautions: high *pitta*.

Osha root is one of the best Western herbs for disorders of the upper respiratory tract, and is therefore commonly used to treat colds, coughs, flu, and viral infections. This hot, pungent tasting herb helps break up the cold and wet qualities of *kapha* in the lungs and GI tract. It works wonderfully for productive coughs to further decongest and expectorate phlegm.

Early spring is predominately a *kapha* time, when its cold, heavy and damp qualities have reached their peak and finely start to thaw, which can contribute to colds and congestive types of disorders, making it a good time to use osha root.

In the Native American tradition, osha is often called "bear root," because it has been observed that bears in the Rocky Mountains seek out and eat it after their long hibernation. This makes perfect sense from an Ayurvedic perspective, since bears have a lot of *kapha* qualities, especially after being in semi-hibernation for several months. They know just what to eat to cleanse and rejuvenate their bodies.

Osha root can often help to ward off a cold or influenza during the first onset, especially when taking other immune supporting and diaphoretic herbs like echinacea, ginger, and *tulsi*. When there is influenza with alternating heat and chills and diminished appetite, it can help to kindle *agni* and burn up *ama*.

In the case of common colds with *pitta* related symptoms, such as yellow, green or bloody sinus mucus, or burning sore throat that continues well beyond the initial stages, then care should be taken to balance osha root with cooling herbs like echinacea, goldenseal, mullein, horehound, licorice, or the Ayurvedic compound *sitopaladi*. A tasty way to soothe a raspy sore throat is to dip a small sprig of the root in licorice powder and chew on it. Osha is a popular addition to cough syrups along with licorice, echinacea, wild cherry bark, and honey, to name a few.

Because many of its properties are not completely water soluble, the tincture is thought to be superior to the tea, although an infusion of the powdered root, in which all the powder is swallowed, makes a strong and effective brew. Osha is a soft root that can be easily pulverized in a mortar and pestle and then ground in an electric coffee grinder.

As a digestive stimulant, it works best for *kapha* and *vata* individuals, who tend to have variable or slow digestive functions.

PEPPERMINT

Mentha piperita; Labiatae

PHUDINA

Effect on Doshas: V+ (in excess) PK-
Rasa: pungent, bitter, sweet **Virya:** slightly cooling **Vipak:** pungent
Preparations: infusion, tincture, oil, salve.
Dosage: 1-30 g per day; tincture, 10-30 drops.

Parts used: aerial portions.

Tissues: plasma, blood, muscle, nerve and marrow.

Systems: digestive, respiratory, nervous, circulatory.

Properties: stimulant, carminative, diaphoretic, nervine, analgesic, antispasmodic.

Indications: indigestion, heartburn, colds, influenza, fever, coughs, sore throat, laryngitis, headaches, dysmenorrhea, flatulence, cramps, colic, sinus congestion, nausea, nervousness, morning sickness, motion sickness, inflammation, colitis, Crohn's disease.

Precautions: high *vata*.

Peppermint soothes digestive complaints and refreshes the mind and nervous system. It is also helpful to reduce excess mucus in the respiratory and GI tracts.

It stimulates the secretion of bile and digestive juices without aggravating *pitta* and is one of the best carminative and antispasmodic herbs, useful in the treatment of colic, flatulence, and dyspepsia. For discomfort associated with irritable or inflammatory bowel disorders, it can be combined with tonic and demulcent herbs like *shatavari*, *vidari*, marshmallow, and licorice.

Care should be taken when using it for chronic weak digestion because its cooling energy may weaken *agni* if used in excess. It is best for *pitta* and *kapha* types of digestive complaints, or as an occasional digestive aid for any constitutional type. It combines well with other carminative herbs such as ginger, fennel, cinnamon, and *ajwan*.

As a cooling diaphoretic, peppermint helps to relieve fevers and other symptoms related to common colds and influenza.

It is also quite effective for relieving headaches caused by increased *pitta*, especially migraines. For this, it can be combined with other cooling nervine herbs like skullcap, gotu kola, or feverfew.

Peppermint essential oil is also effective when applied to the temples for the temporary relief of headaches. A general essential oil blend for headaches can be made by adding equal parts peppermint, sandalwood, rose, and nutmeg oils. A few drops of this mixture can be diluted in a small amount of a base oil, such as sesame or coconut oil, and applied to the temples as needed.

Due to its sweet fragrance, it is frequently used in mouthwashes and toothpastes to freshen the breath. Combined with equal parts fresh ginger, it is a very tasty after dinner tea.

Peppermint helps to reduce anxiety, stress, and nervous tension, although it may increase *vata* when used in excess. That being the case, it is often used in formulation as an assisting or harmonizing herb, rather than given by itself or in large doses.

Pippali

Piper longum; Piperaceae

INDIAN LONG PEPPER

Effect on Doshas: V- P+ K-
Rasa: pungent Virya: heating Vipak: sweet
Preparations: infusion, milk decoction, medicated *ghee*.
Dosage: 1-5 g per day.

Parts used: fruit.

Tissues: plasma, blood, fat, marrow and nerve, reproductive.

Systems: circulatory, digestive, respiratory, nervous, reproductive.

Properties: stimulant, carminative, expectorant, aphrodisiac, analgesic, anthelmintic, rejuvenative.

Indications: colds, influenza, asthma, cough, bronchitis, laryngitis, arthritis, rheumatism, gout, dyspepsia, abdominal distension, flatulence, epilepsy, parasites, worms, obesity, loss of appetite, low metabolism, abdominal tumors, malabsorption, lumbago, poor circulation.

Precautions: high *pitta*, inflammatory conditions.

Pippali is one of the best rejuvenative tonics for the lungs. It has a hot energy yet a sweet post-digestive effect, making it less drying and *pitta* provoking than black pepper, dried ginger, or cayenne. It stimulates *prana agni*, the fire principle present in the respiratory tract, thus increasing vital energy through the breath, and cleansing excess *kapha* and toxins. It is often used to treat common colds, coughs, congestion, and chronic or degenerative lung diseases. It is a key herb in the treatment of asthma and combines well with other lung supportive herbs like *kantakari, tulsi*, or mullein.

Pippali is also a carminative and digestive stimulant used to improve digestion and relieve flatulence and abdominal discomfort. The traditional Ayurvedic wine *pippalyasavam* is used to increase digestive enzymes and is a great remedy for malabsorption, sprue, indigestion, anemia, and loss of appetite.

Pippali is quite effective for improving liver function by stimulating *bhutagni*, the five fire principles in the liver responsible for the transformation of food into the five usable elements that make up our body. Here just 1/4 tsp. of the powder or 1 whole fruit can be taken in the morning with breakfast.

It is often used in the treatment of hepatitis and works to prevent fatty degenerative changes of the liver. A simple remedy to support healthy liver function can be made by mixing 1/4 tsp. of the ground fruit with 1/2 tsp. of *ghee* and 1 tsp. raw honey, and eaten daily first thing in the morning, followed by warm water. This mixture is also good for those who have recently quit smoking to cleanse and rejuvenate damaged and toxic lung tissue. Eating one pippali fruit a day is also good to support normal thyroid function.

Because it helps to control *vata* and *kapha* and to burn *ama*, it is used for rheumatoid arthritis (*ama vata*), a condition caused by *vata* pushing *ama* into the joints. A good home remedy for *ama vata* can be made by combining 1/4 tsp. each of pippali and ginger powder and 1 tsp. of castor oil in 1 cup of hot water and taken before bedtime daily.

A medicated milk preparation for rejuvenating the lungs made with this herb is called *pippali siddhadugdha*. It is prepared by adding 5 whole fruits or 1/2 tsp. of the powder to 1 cup of whole milk and 1/2 cup of water, boiling it in a covered pot until only 1 cup of liquid remains. The decoction is then strained and taken first thing in the morning. This same preparation can be enhanced by increasing the quantity of whole fruits each day by one until a total of 64 fruits are used and then decreasing one each day until only 5 remain. For this method, only the whole fruits are used, not the powder. This practice is considered to have profound physical benefits, as well as the spiritual bonus of enhancing one's *sattwic* nature.

Poke Root

Phytolacca spp; Phytolaccaceae

Effect on Doshas: V+ PK-
Rasa: bitter Virya: cooling Vipak: pungent
Preparations: infusion, decoction, poultices, fresh root oil.
Dosage: 250 mg-1 g per day; tincture, 1-5 drops per day.

Parts used: root.

Tissues: plasma, blood, fat.

Systems: lymphatic, respiratory, urinary, immune.

Properties: alterative, anti-tumor, anti-rheumatic, anodyne, purgative, emetic, catarrhal.

Indications: glandular and lymphatic swellings, mastitis, tumors, cysts, breast cancer, rheumatism, scabies, antiviral, antiseptic, respiratory tract infections, pneumonia, skin diseases, goiter.

Precautions: Most every part of this plant is toxic and should be used with much care. It can cause rashes when used topically, and nausea and diarrhea in medium to high doses. Avoid in cases of high *vata* and pregnancy.

Poke root has a powerful cleansing action upon the blood and lymphatic tissues. It is pacifying to *pitta* and *kapha* and has an affinity to the throat, lungs, breasts, ovaries, and uterus. It helps to boost the immune system and is effective for the treatment of acute as well as chronic infections. It has proven to be quite useful for treating tonsillitis, laryngitis, swollen glands, goiter, and mastitis, while it also helps to remove excess phlegm from the upper respiratory tract.

It clears excess *kapha* in the form of lymphatic congestion, cysts and tumors, making it quite useful in the treatment of fibrocystic changes of the breasts and in some cases of breast cancer. An infused oil of poke root can be applied topically for reducing breast lumps although the oil may be irritating to the skin and may cause a rash in some people. There are many documented cases of successful treatment of breast cancer with salves, extracts, and poultices containing poke root, but such treatment is often not an easy process and must be overseen by a highly skilled practitioner with experience in these procedures.

Poke root helps in the reduction of *ama* and is a valuable remedy for treating chronic rheumatic conditions. Because it is such a powerful detoxifying herb, it should be used with caution and along with other herbs as a part of a holistic treatment. For internal use I suggest using it in small doses ranging from 1 to 5 drops per day.

Prickly Ash

Xanthoxylum americanum; Rutaceae

Effect on Doshas: V- P+ K-
Rasa: pungent, bitter Virya: heating Vipak: pungent
Preparations: infusion, decoction, liniment, medicated oil, tincture.
Dosage: 2-5 g per day; tincture, 10-30 drops.

Parts used: bark and berries.

Tissues: plasma, blood, muscle, fat.

Systems: digestive, circulatory.

Properties: stimulant, carminative, alterative, antibacterial, antiseptic, anthelmintic, analgesic.

Indications: cold hands and feet, abdominal distention and discomfort, chills, arthritis, rheumatism, yeast infections, worms, slow or variable digestion, dental problems, Raynaud's disease, arteriosclerosis, dry mouth.

Precautions: high *pitta*, pregnancy, acute inflammatory conditions of the GI tract.

Prickly Ash is stimulating to the peripheral circulation and is commonly used for cold extremities, cramps, chilblains, varicose veins, and rheumatism. It is used to correct excess *vata* and *kapha*, and to help kindle *agni*, burn *ama*, and relieve gas, bloating, and abdominal discomfort.

To clear excess heat, neutralize toxins, and soothe irritated mucous membranes for *pitta* related digestive conditions, it combines well with more cooling herbs like gentian, oregon grape root, and licorice.

It works well as an antibacterial mouthwash for treating gingivitis, canker sores, receding gums, bad breath, toothaches, and bleeding gums. For this, it can be mixed with other antiseptic or astringent herbs like bayberry bark, *neem* bark, echinacea, and *bilva*. These herbs can be made into a tooth powder for brushing or a tincture, which can be diluted with a little distilled water and used as a mouth wash.

Topically, prickly ash can be used in a stimulating liniment or prepared along with other herbs as a massage oil for inflamed and arthritic conditions.

Punarnava

Boerhaavia diffusa; Nyctaginaceae

Effect on Doshas: V+ (in excess) PK-
Rasa: bitter, sweet, pungent, slightly astringent **Virya:** cooling **Vipak:** pungent
Preparations: infusion, decoction, paste, eye drops (or wash).
Dosage: 1-9 g per day.

Parts used: aerial portions, roots.

Tissues: plasma, blood, fat, marrow and nerve, reproductive.

Systems: digestive, urinary, nervous, reproductive, respiratory, circulatory.

Properties: diuretic, diaphoretic, laxative, rejuvenative, alterative, emetic, expectorant, bitter tonic.

Indications: edema, obesity, heart disease, eye diseases, skin diseases, rheumatism, urinary tract conditions, kidney and bladder stones, gallstones, hemorrhoids, asthma, hypertension, respiratory disorders, arthritis, gout, prostate disorders, fibrocystic changes, cysts, tumors, jaundice, hepatitis, gonorrhea, snake and rat bites.

Precautions: high *vata*, dehydration, low kidney energy.

Punarnava is one of the most respected and widely used *kapha* reducing herbs in Ayurvedic medicine. It pacifies *pitta* and *kapha* and has an affinity to the kidneys, heart, lungs, eyes, and liver. It is used for coughs, bronchitis, *kapha* type of asthma, glaucoma, rheumatism, gout, skin diseases, piles, edema, obesity and heart related disorders.

It is a cooling diuretic, so it helps to relieve excess heat from the system, while also cooling and soothing mucous membranes. It cleanses the kidneys and urinary tract and helps to discharge urinary or gallstones. To treat urinary tract infections, it is good combined with herbs like *gokshura, shatavari, guduchi*, uva ursi, and pipsissewa.

Punarnava is rich in potassium salts, especially potassium nitrate, and will not deplete the body like many conventional diuretic medicines do. However, if a diuretic is needed and there is general low energy and fatigue, then it is best used along with *gokshura*, which tends to be more nourishing and rejuvenating.

When designing formulas to balance *kapha*, punarnava is one of the best choices because it helps to bring excess *kleda*, the liquid component of *kapha*, from almost any part of the body toward the kidneys and urinary tract to be eliminated. Combining it with a *yogavahi* (catalytic agent) can help to direct and enhance its diuretic action upon a specific region of the body. For example, when addressing the heart, it combines well with *arjuna* or elecampane; for the joints with *guggulu*; and for the lungs with mullein, red clover, *pippali*, or *kantakari*. It can make an effective addition to formulas used to treat hypertension, especially caused by *kapha* or *pitta*.

Punarnava has also proven useful for the treatment of hepatitis and fatty degenerative changes in the liver, as well as skin diseases such as eczema and psoriasis. For this, it combines well with liver supporting herbs like *kutki* or gentian, milk thistle, burdock, dandelion, *neem*, or *shankapushpi*.

For treating asthma and other congestive respiratory complaints, it helps to clear excess *kapha* from the lungs and can be mixed with expectorating and bronchodilating herbs like *kantakari* and *pippali*, and herbs that liquefy phlegm such as licorice or comfrey root.

A general formula to burn fat, increase the metabolism, and reduce and prevent abnormal accumulations of tissues (such as fibrocystic breasts, lipomas, and cysts) can be made by combining 5 parts punarnava to 3 parts *chitrak*, 3 parts red clover and 2 parts each of *kutki* (or gentian) and *trikatu*. This mixture can be taken in doses of 1 tsp. in hot water with raw honey, 3 times daily, after meals.

Punarnava eye drops or eyewash have shown to be quite effective for treating glaucoma and cataracts. For this, an infusion can be made by adding 1/4 tsp. each punarnava and *triphala* in hot water and letting it steep till it has cooled. Strain it well through a coffee filter or cheesecloth and apply using a glass eyewash cup. This can be done 1 to 2 times daily. To rejuvenate the eyes, it can be combined with equal parts *shatavari*.

Punarnava is the main herb in the Ayurvedic formula *punarnavadi guggulu*, which is used, amongst other conditions, for arthritis (especially with swelling), edema, obesity, and kidney and urinary disorders.

Red Raspberry Leaf

Rubus spp.; Rosaceae

Effect on Doshas: V+ (in excess) PK-
Rasa: mildly bitter, astingent, sweet **Virya:** cooling **Vipak:** sweet
Preparations: infusion, tincture, paste.
Dosage: 6-15 g per day.

Parts used: leaves, berries.

Tissues: plasma, blood, muscle, bone, reproductive.

Systems: digestive, female reproductive, urinary.

Properties: astringent, alterative, tonic, hemostatic, antiemetic.

Indications: diarrhea, dysentery, cankers, gingivitis, nausea, vomiting, uterine bleeding, menorrhagia, dysmenorrhea, prolapsed uterus or anus, inflammation of mucous membranes, ulcers, gastritis, heart burn, sore throat, to prevent miscarriage.

Precautions: high *vata*.

Raspberry leaf is primarily a *pitta* and *kapha* pacifying herb with astringent and mild tonic properties and affinities to the uterus, colon, and the entire genitourinary tract. It can provoke *vata* when used in excess, so to prevent this it is best used with stronger tonic herbs like *shatavari* and *vidari*.

It is well known as a prenatal tonic to nourish and support the womb in preparation for childbirth, ease of labor, and to prevent miscarriage. For this, it can be combined with a more rejuvenative tonic herb like *shatavari*. It is best used only in the last trimester of pregnancy for those women who are either *vata* types or underweight.

After childbirth, it can be used to regain the tone of the female reproductive organs and is effectively used in the treatment of prolapsed uterus or anus, uterine hemorrhage, profuse menstrual flow, hemorrhoids, and to regulate the menstrual cycle. Being a rich source in iron, manganese, and niacin, it helps to replenish the blood and strengthen the connective tissues. It is therefore useful to treat anemia, for which it combines well with *amalaki* or nettles.

Its astringent and *pitta* soothing effect on the GI tract helps in cases of diarrhea, dysentery, heartburn, ulcers, and nausea. A douche of the tea can also relieve vaginal inflammation, itching, irritation, and prolapse.

Raspberry leaf tea can also be used as a mouthwash or gargle for canker sores, gingivitis, and sore throats, or applied topically to promote healing of burns and wounds.

RED CLOVER

Trifolium pratense; Leguminasae

VANA-METHIKA

Effect on Doshas: V+ (in excess) PK-
Rasa: bitter, sweet **Virya:** cooling **Vipak:** pungent
Preparations: infusion, tincture, paste.
Dosage: 6-15 g per day; tincture, 30-60 drops.

Parts used: blossoms and leaves.

Tissues: plasma, blood, bone, reproductive.

Systems: circulatory, lymphatic, reproductive.

Properties: alterative, antispasmodic, expectorant, anti-tumor, diuretic.

Indications: skin eruptions, coughs, colds, congestion, bronchitis, cancer, infections, degenerative disorders.

Precautions: Hemophiliacs or people with thin blood should not use red clover on a regular basis because of the presence of coumarins in the plant, which have blood thinning properties.

Red clover is rich in nitrogen and minerals, including calcium, iron, potassium, chromium, and magnesium, as well as phosphorus and vitamins like niacin, thiamine, and vitamin C. It is a gentle and effective blood tonic and purifier and is helpful for treating *pitta* related skin diseases such as eczema, psoriasis, and boils. It is fairly *tridoshic* although it may increase *vata* if used in large amounts or for extended periods.

Many alterative herbs are often too cold and depleting to *vata* types, young children, and the elderly, but red clover is an exception to the rule and is good for sensitive or weak individuals that may benefit from a blood cleansing, bitter herb.

Due to its mild antispasmodic and expectorant qualities, it can relieve chronic coughs and bronchial congestion. For sinus or respiratory tract infections, it combines well with *pitta* reducing herbs such as mullein, coltsfoot, and horehound to help clear excess heat and dampness.

In Western herbalism, red clover has proven to be an invaluable herb in the treatment of breast cancer and fibrocystic breast changes, and is used to soften and reduce cysts, tumors, and cancerous growths. It is the leading herb in the Western herbal compound known as Hoxsey's formula, which is held in high regard for supporting the treatment of breast cancer.

A warm fomentation of red clover can be applied to the breast tissue, and kept warm with a hot water bottle, to break up abnormal growths or relieve tenderness.

As an herbal paste or tea, it can be applied locally to minor cuts, burns, and abrasions to promote healing.

Shankapushpi

Evolvulus alsinoides; Convolvulaceae

DWARF MORNING GLORY

Effect on Doshas: VPK=
Rasa: bitter, pungent, astringent **Virya:** cooling **Vipak:** sweet
Preparations: infusion, decoction, syrups, medicated *ghee*, milk decoction, paste.
Dosage: 3-12 g per day.

Parts used: aerial portions.

Tissues: plasma, blood, fat, marrow and nerve, reproductive.

Systems: digestive, circulatory, urinary, nervous.

Properties: alterative, nervine, vulnerary, bitter tonic, aphrodisiac, diuretic, hemostatic.

Indications: liver diseases, sluggish liver function, skin diseases, toxicity, ADD, nervous disorders, depression, psychosis, epilepsy, memory loss, insomnia, jaundice, low libido, gallstones, anxiety, indigestion, dysentery, fever, possession, nervous debility, speech impediments.

Shankapushpi is one of the best rejuvenative herbs for the mind and nervous system. It pacifies all three *doshas* and is often given along with other *medhya rasayana* (mental rejuvenative) herbs like gotu kola, *brahmi, jatamansi*, and calamus (*vacha*). It corrects aggravated *vata* and is helpful in cases of nervous debility, depression, epilepsy, psychosis, ADD, memory loss, and insomnia. The freshly extracted juice of the plant has the strongest action, although the dried herb is what is typically available in the West and works quite well.

It purifies the *raktavaha srotas* (blood channel), making it useful for treating skin diseases like eczema and psoriasis. For this type of condition, it can also be applied locally as a medicated *ghee*.

It is a key herb for protecting and rejuvenating the liver, so it can very helpful for chronic hepatitis and cirrhosis. Here it is often used in combination with other blood cleansing herbs such as *guduchi, neem*, *kutki*, gentian, or milk thistle.

Due to its mild hemostatic properties, it can help to stop bleeding in the GI, reproductive, and urinary tracts.

Shankapushpi is also a valuable remedy for dysentery, constipation, indigestion, and fevers accompanied by diarrhea and indigestion.

For reproductive issues, it can be made as a milk decoction along with herbs like *ashwagandha, shatavari*, and kapi kacchu to promote fertility in both men and women.

It can be burned as incense to cleanse and purify the atmosphere of negative energies and to purify the subtle body.

Shatavari

Asparagus racemosus; Liliaceae

ASPARAGUS ROOT

Effect on Doshas: VP- K+
Rasa: bitter, sweet **Virya:** cooling **Vipak:** sweet
Preparations: infusion, decoction, powder, paste, jam, milk decoction, medicated *ghee.*
Dosage: 3-30 g per day.

Parts used: root.

Tissues: acts upon all tissues.

Systems: reproductive, circulatory. respiratory, digestive, urinary.

Properties: alterative, demulcent, nutritive tonic, rejuvenative, mild diuretic, anti-inflammatory, galactagogue, aphrodisiac.

Indications: female reproductive disorders, leucorrhea, scanty breast milk flow, sexual debility, infertility, impotence, menopause, diarrhea, dysentery, hyperacidity, ulcers, colitis, gastritis, dehydration, lung abscess, hematemesis, dry cough, cancer, herpes, chronic fevers, excessive thirst, fatigue, convalescence.

Precautions: high *kapha* and *ama*, excessive mucus.

In Sanskrit, *Shatavari* means "she who possesses a hundred husbands," due to its ability to increase fertility and nourish the ovum. Although often thought of as a women's herb, its reproductive action extends to men as well.

It is one of the primary *rasayanas* for *pitta* and is rejuvenative to the entire female reproductive system. It also has an affinity to the blood, liver, kidneys, lungs, and the entire GI tract.

It possesses hormone-like properties and helps to regulate the menstrual cycle. It is specific for *pitta* related menstrual disorders, characterized by profuse menstrual bleeding, painful burning, and irritation.

Shatavari is also an effective herb used to ease the transition into menopause, especially when combined with equal parts *vidari* or wild yam. One tsp. of this mixture can be taken with warm water 3 times a day.

In cases of hysterectomy, shatavari can help to restore balance at an emotional and energetic level when combined with *brahmi* or *jatamansi*.

It also helps to improve the quantity and quality of breast milk and to nourish the fetus when taken during pregnancy. For weakness during pregnancy, 1/2 tsp. of a mixture of equal parts shatavari and *ashwagandha* can be taken with warm water 1-2 times a day to bolster energy and balance *vata*.

Its cooling and demulcent properties can soothe inflamed mucous membranes throughout the entire GI tract, kidneys, and urinary tract, as well as the reproductive system. Therefore, it is used in the treatment of disorders such as hyperacidity, diarrhea, gastritis, colitis, ulcers, and urinary tract infections.

Shatavari is often used as a leading herb in constitutionally based formulas for *pitta* predominant individuals and/or *pitta* imbalances. When there is high *kapha* or *ama* present, then similar but lighter herbs, such as *guduchi* or burdock, can be used in its place. Western asparagus root has a similar action but is more diuretic and less of a tonic.

Having both sweet and bitter tastes and a sweet post-digestive effect (*vipak*), it is a good blood purifying herb to choose for *vata* types or for those in a weakened or debilitated state, because it is not drying and depleting, like many alterative herbs can be. Qualitatively, it inhibits the dry, light, rough, and mobile qualities of *vata*, and is a nourishing and strengthening tonic.

Shatavari rasayana is a simple formula for promoting overall health of the female reproductive tissue and the flow and quality of breast milk. It can be made by toasting 4 parts shatavari, 2 parts *ghee*, 2 parts sugar, 1/3 part cardamom and a pinch of saffron in a cast iron pan on a low heat, stirring continuously until the mixture is slightly browned. The quantity of the *ghee* can be varied to change the consistency. The dosage for this *rasayana* is 1 tsp. twice daily with warm milk or water.

Another recipe that can be used in much the same way is a shatavari milk decoction, which consists of 1 tsp. of shatavari boiled in 1 cup of milk along with a pinch of saffron and cardamom, and 1 tsp. each of raw sugar and *ghee*. This milk decoction can be taken daily, first thing in the morning, on an empty stomach.

Shatavari medicated *ghee* is also rejuvenating to the reproductive system. It aids with lactation and promotes the growth of the breast tissue. Daily breast massage with the ghee, especially during early stages of breast development, can promote optimal breast growth. When taken internally, it also helps to kindle *agni*, protect *ojas*, increase immunity, and to treat chronic fatigue and inflammatory bowel disorders such as Crohn's disease and ulcerative colitis.

Shilajit

Asphaltum punjabianum

MINERAL PITCH

Effect on Doshas: V- P+ (in excess) K-
Rasa: pungent, bitter, salty, astringent Virya: heating Vipak: pungent
Preparations: liquid form, pill.
Dosage: 250 mg-5 g per day.

Parts used: mineral pitch.

Tissues: works on all tissues.

Systems: urinary, reproductive, nervous, circulatory.

Properties: diuretic, rejuvenative tonic, nervine, sedative, alterative, anthelmintic, anti-microbial, lithotriptic, aphrodisiac.

Indications: anemia, asthma, bronchitis, kidney and urinary disorders, cystitis, obesity, edema, diabetes, glycosuria, general debility, fatigue, menorrhagia, dysmenorrhea, seminal debility, low sexual energy, enlarged prostate, enlarged spleen, nocturnal emission, premature ejaculation, spermatorrhea, spermaturia, gallstones and kidney stones, high cholesterol, nervous debility, epilepsy.

Precautions: high *pitta*, use with care during pregnancy.

Shilajit is a Sanskrit word meaning "conqueror of mountains and destroyer of weakness." It is a black tar-like mineral pitch that exudes from certain rocks in the Himalayan regions, in the summer season, and forms as a result of the decomposing vegetation. There are several types of shilajit, such as black, red, gold, white, and blue, but in general it is the black variety that is used for medicinal purposes. It is an indispensable medicine in Ayurveda, revered as being able to treat a wide array of diseases. It is a rich source of minerals in ionic form, such as magnesium, zinc, iron, and silica, as well as humic acid and fulvic acid. It helps to build *rakta dhatu* (blood) and *asthi dhatu* (bone).

Because of its heating, drying, and scraping action, it helps to balance *kapha*, but in excess it may be too heating to *pitta* and reducing to *vata*. For this reason, it needs to be used with care and is often taken along with other tonic herbs. Furthermore, even though it is nourishing to the bodily tissues, it should be used with caution in wasting types of conditions due to excess *vata* in the muscle and fat tissues.

Shilajit is a rejuvenative to the kidneys, urinary tract, reproductive and immune systems, as well as the lungs. It helps to regulate *apana vayu* and is used for reproductive disorders such as infertility and sterility, dysmenorrhea associated with high *vata*, urinary diseases, and diabetes.

Its powerful *kapha* managing properties make it useful for breaking down and flushing out kidney and gallstones, and reducing high cholesterol and obesity.

In the case of adult on-set diabetes, it combines well with *neem* and turmeric to control blood sugar levels and to prevent weight gain.

For under active thyroid function, it can be formulated with *guduchi* or *kaishore guggulu*.

Shilajit is a far better choice than viagra, due to its ability to increase virility and sexual stamina while maintaining the normal tone of the genital organs. For this, it is best combined with *ashwagandha* in a ratio of 1 to 3.

For enlarged prostate it can be helpful alone or along with *gokshuradi guggulu*, *ashwagandha*, saw palmetto, or *vidari*.

SKULLCAP

Scutellaria lateriflora; Labiatae

Effect on Doshas: V+ (in excess) PK-
Rasa: bitter Virya: cooling Vipak: pungent
Preparations: infusion, tincture, *nasya*.
Dosage: 1-9 g per day; tincture, 30-60 drops.

Parts used: aerial portions.

Tissues: plasma, blood, marrow and nerve, reproductive.

Systems: nervous, circulatory.

Properties: nervine tonic, sedative, antispasmodic, alterative.

Indications: nervous tension, insomnia, stress, anxiety, neurosis, neuralgia, emotional disturbances, seizures, spasms, tremors, addictions, hysteria, recovery, PMS, hypertension.

Precautions: high *vata*.

Skullcap works exceptionally well to relax and replenish the nervous system, thus relieving stress, nervous tension, anxiety, and worry. It is a calming herb that can be used as a *vata* and nerve tonic, and can be combined with more nourishing tonic herbs such as *ashwagandha* or *bala*. It has also shown to be valuable at relieving premenstrual symptoms.

Being a cooling nervine, it is usually used for insomnia caused by an overdriven, over stimulated *pitta* mind. It helps to let go of the day without the heaviness caused by more grounding sedatives. For general stress and restlessness, it combines well with chamomile, and for insomnia with restlessness in the body and mind, it works well with valerian for *vata* types or with cooling nervine herbs like *hops* or chamomile for *pitta* individuals.

Skullcap helps to restore the balance of *sadhaka pitta*, the subtype of *pitta* responsible for the functions of the intellect, memory, comprehension, enthusiasm, and higher mind functions. It is also a mild blood purifying herb that helps to dispel excess *pitta* from the general circulation.

It is a *medhya rasayana*, a brain tonic, and has a *sattwic* quality that helps to promote clarity, awareness, and one pointed concentration. To enhance meditation, it can be combined with equal parts gotu kola and taken as a warm infusion in 1 tsp. size doses per cup, an hour before meditating.

It helps to purify the *nadis* (subtle energy pathways), for which it combines well with equal parts calamus (*vacha*).

It has an affinity to the heart chakra and can be combined with other herbs that act directly upon the heart like *arjuna* or elecampane to help resolve deep seated emotional blocks that have become lodged in the *hridaya dhara kala* (pericardium).

For emotional imbalances caused by increased *pitta*, such as anger, criticism, and irritability, it can be combined with equal parts gotu kola, chamomile, and licorice.

Skullcap has proven useful in easing the detoxification during recovery from alcohol or barbiturate abuse, especially when taken in small frequent doses (10-20 drops of the tincture).

St. John's Wort

Hypericum perforatum; Hypericaceae

Effect on Doshas: V+ (in excess) PK-
Rasa: bitter, sweet Virya: cooling Vipak: pungent
Preparations: infusion, poultice, salves and lotions, simple oil infusion of the fresh flower in olive oil.
Dosage: 3-9 g per day; tincture, 10-60 drops.

Parts used: aerial portions.

Tissues: plasma, blood, nerve and marrow.

Systems: nervous, digestive, respiratory.

Properties: nervine sedative and tonic, analgesic, anti-inflammatory, anti- depressant, antiviral, antispasmodic, expectorant, astringent.

Indications: mild to moderate depression, stress, nervous tension, spasms, muscle cramps, neuralgia, rheumatism, sciatica, nerve damage, inflammation, bruises, minor wounds.

Precautions: possibly high *vata* if used alone in large doses for extended periods of time, although when used in formulation it can be quite beneficial to *vata* conditions of the nervous system.

Saint John's Wort has been used for centuries in Western European herbal traditions as a nervine tonic, sedative, and analgesic herb. Taken both internally or applied topically as a liniment or oil, it helps to relieve neuromuscular and rheumatic pain, as well as shifting or migrating pain, which is often associated with the erratic, mobile qualities of *vata dosha*.

It aids in the healing of minor burns and wounds and is a common ingredient in healing lotions and salves along with other vulnerary herbs like comfrey, plantain, or calendula.

When used in moderation, St. John's Wort is fairly *tridoshic* and can act as a buffer to general stress, easing emotional factors that tend to accompany many *doshic* imbalances, thus making the person more receptive to any healing process.

It has a rejuvenating effect on the mind and nervous system and is effective in the treatment of mild to moderate forms of depression. For *vata* types of depression, characterized by fear, anxiety, worry, and restlessness, it combines well with nourishing and nutritive tonics like *ashwagandha, bala, dashamula,* and calming herbs like *jatamansi*, avena, chamomile, and *shankapushpi.*

For *pitta* types of emotional disturbances associated with anger, rage, and irritability, it can be combined with herbs like gotu kola, skullcap, *bhringaraj*, *shankapushpi*, rose petals, or lemon balm.

Kapha types of depression can often be accompanied by the urge to hold on and become severely attached to others. This can manifest in the desire to seek love and satisfaction through the sweet taste. Here it works well with *shardunika* to reduce sweet cravings and with aromatic digestive herbs like ginger, *vacha* (calamus), cardamom, and clove.

Because of its affinity to the nerve tissue, St. John's Wort is useful for trauma to the spine, head, or any other nerve rich areas like the tips of the toes or fingers.

It has antiviral properties and helps to clear excess *pitta* from the blood and the nervous system. It is quite useful for the treatment of herpes and shingles and their associated emotional components. For this, it is often used with herbs like *neem*, licorice, turmeric, *manjista*, and echinacea.

It is a *sattwic* herb that helps to promote awareness, clarity, and relaxation and makes a good tea for supporting meditation. The fresh flowers contain a lot of solar energy and help to bring a similar sense of joy and peace that sunshine does, making it a nice herb to consider for seasonal depression during the winter or rainy seasons.

TULSI, TULASI

Ocimum sanctum; Lamiaceae

HOLY BASIL

Effect on Doshas: V- P+ (in excess) K-
Rasa: pungent, bitter, astringent Virya: heating Vipak: pungent
Preparations: infusion, paste, fresh juice, medicated *ghee*, tincture.
Dosage: 1-12 g per day; tincture, 30-60 drops.

Parts used: leaves, seeds, stems, root.

Tissues: plasma, blood, muscle, marrow and nerve, reproductive.

Systems: respiratory, urinary, nervous, circulatory, digestive

Properties: demulcent, expectorant, diaphoretic, febrifuge, antiseptic, antibacterial, anthelmintic, nervine, sedative, adaptogen, diuretic.

Indications: asthma, colds, cough, sinus congestion, bronchitis, fevers, influenza, headaches, stress, sore throat, tonsillitis, kidney stones, heart disorders, stress, mouth infections, arthritis, rheumatism, abdominal distention, boils, skin diseases, dysentery, colitis, diarrhea, earache, parasites, snake and insect bites.

Precautions: *nirama pitta*.

Tulsi is a native plant to India that is now grown in many regions throughout the world. There are mainly two varieties of tulsi: Rama or Krishna Tulsi (*Ocimum sanctum*) and Vana Tulsi (*Ocimum gratissimum*) and a variety of *Ocimum tenuiflorum* used in Thai cuisine, which is referred to as Thai holy basil, or *kha phrao*—not be confused with Thai basil, which is a variety of the sweet, common *Ocimum basilicum*.

Tulsi leaves are highly aromatic, especially when fresh. The medicinal and spiritual uses of this sacred plant date back thousands of years, to the ancient Vedic period. *Tulsi*, which is Sanskrit for "the incomparable one," is worshiped throughout India, most often regarded as a manifestation of the Goddess Vrindavani, or as the consort of Vishnu in the form of Mahalakshmi. It is commonly grown in or around Hindu homes and temples to purify and sanctify the atmosphere. The leaves are also used in daily worship of Vishnu, Rama, and Krishna. The woody stem is made into prayer beads, which, when worn or used for chanting, can open the heart, increase *sattwic* tendencies like *bhakti* (devotion), and promote health and longevity.

It is thought to aid in the release of deep-seated emotions, such as grief and sadness lodged in the pericardium and lungs. The warm tea with a little honey, first thing in the morning, helps to refresh the mind, nourish the respiratory and nervous systems, and can also aid in lowering cholesterol. The fresh leaves can also be chewed or taken as a tea to reduce stress and stimulate *sadhaka pitta*, thus promoting intelligence.

For headaches caused by stress, it can be applied to the forehead as a paste made with equal parts sandalwood powder and a little aloe vera juice or water.

Tulsi helps to strengthen the heart and acts as a coronary vasodilator, thus promoting oxygenation of the heart muscle. As a general heart tonic, it combines well with equal parts *arjuna* and can be taken with honey. The mixture made into a paste can also be taken orally in small frequent doses for relieving angina pectoris.

It is commonly used to dispel phlegm from the respiratory tract and is effective in the treatment of asthma, cough, bronchitis, and sinus congestion. For acute asthma, combine it with herbs like mullein, *pippali*, and lobelia. It also has diaphoretic and febrifuge properties that help in treating fever due to the common cold and flu, by burning *ama* and inducing sweating. Its pleasant taste makes it easy for children to tolerate in such conditions.

Its diuretic and antibacterial properties make tulsi useful for kidney related conditions, including nephritis, kidney stones, and bladder infections. For this, consider combining it with other diuretic herbs like *punarnava* or *gokshura*. An infusion of the fresh or dried leaves can be given in cases of malaria and liver disorders. Its recurrent use has proven useful to regulate blood sugar levels.

Tulsi helps to mitigate excess *vata* in the GI tract and promotes absorption. It makes a tasty digestive tea when combined with fresh ginger, cardamom, and fennel and is great for intestinal colic in infants and children.

Its seeds are demulcent and cooling and more *pitta* pacifying than the leaves. They can be used to correct diarrhea, cystitis, and high fever.

For healing ulcerative colitis, the seeds are soaked overnight in cool water, then strained and added to 1/2 cup of fresh yogurt.

A few of the fresh leaves mixed with 1/4 tsp. of rock candy powder and eaten daily, first thing in the morning, can be a useful remedy for relieving nausea due to high *pitta*.

When the leaf is mixed with lime juice, it is extremely effective for certain skin diseases, including ringworm, scabies, and leprosy. In this case, it can also be mixed with *neem*.

An effective home remedy for earaches in children consists in applying a few drops of the fresh leaf juice in the ear twice a day until the pain is gone. The leaves can also be used in the preparation of garlic oil, which can be very helpful for ear infections, tinnitus, hearing loss, and general earaches.

Simply gargling with tulsi tea helps to soothe a sore throat, heal gum infection, and freshen the breath.

TURMERIC

Curcuma longa; Zingiberaceae

HARIDRA, HALDI

Effect on Doshas: V-P+ (in excess) K-
Rasa: bitter, pungent, astringent **Virya:** heating **Vipak:** pungent
Preparations: infusion, decoction, milk decoction, paste, tincture, *ghee.*
Dosage: 1-9 g per day; tincture, 30-60 drops.

Parts used: rhizome.

Tissues: acts upon all tissues.

Systems: digestive, circulatory, respiratory, urinary.

Properties: stimulant, carminative, cholagogue, alterative, anti-inflammatory, vulnerary, antibacterial, anthelmintic, antiviral, antibiotic, tonic.

Indications: colds, coughs, sore throat, pharyngitis, asthma, allergies, infections, poor circulation, diabetes, arthritis, anemia, wounds, bruises, skin disorders, weak digestion, indigestion, sprains.

Precautions: high *pitta*, pregnancy, acute jaundice and hepatitis.

Turmeric is probably one of the most common cooking spices in Indian cuisine and is an invaluable medicinal herb used in Ayurveda. It enhances metabolic energy and helps to digest proteins, especially legumes. In fact, there are very few bean dishes in Indian cooking where turmeric is not found. It is a natural preservative, thus preventing food from spoiling too quickly when cooked with it.

It is supportive to healthy liver function, thereby detoxifying the blood. As a natural antibiotic, it is used to treat all sorts of infections and inflammatory conditions without disturbing the intestinal flora. It helps to cleanse and improve the overall terrain of the GI tract. Its tonic and immune supporting properties make it a good medicine for chronic weakness or illness.

For skin disorders like acne, urticaria, eczema, and psoriasis, it combines well with other alterative herbs like Oregon grape root, burdock, *manjista*, *neem*, and *guduchi*. A small amount of the powdered herb can be mixed into a little *neem* oil and applied topically to rashes to relief itching. This remedy is also very effective for fungal infections of the skin and nails.

For fungal infections of the nails, where the nail becomes detached from its nail bed, turmeric tincture is most effective because it penetrates under the nail easier than when combined with a base oil. In some cases, after several months of daily use of the tincture, the infected nail reattaches and grows back as good as new. I have personally seen this work remarkably well when used every day without fail.

Turmeric has an affinity to the lungs and can be used for the treatment of asthma, bronchial congestion, and allergies. For this, it combines well with other immune tonic herbs like *guduchi*, nettles, and *amalaki*. A general lung tonic can be made by boiling 1 tsp. of the dried powder in a cup of milk and taken first thing in the morning or before bedtime.

Its antiseptic and astringent properties make it useful in first aid for disinfecting open wounds (especially when mixed with raw honey) and to stop bleeding.

For sore throat, a nice remedy is to gargle with a mixture made by stirring well 1 tsp. of turmeric with 1/2 tsp. sea salt in a cup of warm water.

Turmeric makes a great poultice to suppurate boils as well. A simple recipe for this can be made by lightly steaming a good chunk of fresh onion, then mashing it along with 1 tsp. of turmeric powder, making it into a semi thick paste that can be applied locally and wrapped in gauze.

Even though turmeric has a warming energy, it helps to reduce inflammation in muscles and tendons due to its *prabhava*, or special action. From a Western perspective, turmeric is thought to inhibit the synthesis of prostaglandins in the body that are associated with pain, as well as to stimulate the adrenal glands to release their own cortisone, a potent pain reliever. It has also shown to be effective in the treatment of bursitis, tendonitis, and arthritis, as well as for traumatic injuries.

For sprains, mix equal parts turmeric powder and sea salt, and add enough hot water to make a thick paste. Apply it to the injured part, wrap it well, and prop up the limb to rest. This will help to reduce the swelling, pain, and inflammation, as well as to promote a speedy recovery. Be aware that the skin will turn yellow for some time, but it is worth it. It can also be mixed with honey for sprains and strains.

According to Ayurveda, treating injured joints with ice packs should only be done as a first aid and within the first 24 hours of the injury, and then contrasted with warmth to promote circulation. Too much ice therapy can predispose the joint to reinjury or to arthritic changes in the future.

For conjunctivitis, a cold infusion of the powder can be used as an eyewash twice daily.

Taking turmeric regularly as a spice in the daily diet helps to inhibit the accumulation of metabolic waste products, to relieve flatulence, and to prevent gallstone formation. Recent studies have shown that regular use of turmeric may be beneficial for the treatment and prevention of certain cancers, as well.

Turmeric has a *sattwic* quality and is purifying to the *nadis* (subtle energy channels). It is thought to bestow the energy of the divine mother and is often used to color white rice to be used as a symbolic offering in Vedic religious ceremonies.

Uva Ursi

Arctostaphylos uva ursi; Ericaceae

Effect on Doshas: V+ PK-
Rasa: bitter, astringent Virya: cooling Vipak: pungent
Preparations: infusion, decoction, tincture.
Dosage: 3-9 g per day; tincture, 30-60 drops.

Parts used: leaves.

Tissues: blood, plasma.

Systems: urinary.

Properties: antiseptic, diuretic, astringent.

Indications: cystitis, nephritis, urethritis, hematuria, pyelitis, healing of minor wounds.

Precautions: high *vata*, sensitive stomach.

Uva ursi, also known as bearberry, has been used for hundreds of years as a remedy for urinary tract infections. Native Americans used it as a medicinal plant for that purpose and, in fact, until the discovery of sulfa drugs and antibiotics, uva ursi was the most common treatment for bladder and related infections.

It is a urinary antiseptic that is very effective in treating high *pitta* conditions by cooling mucous membranes of the urinary tract and is used for disorders like cystitis, vaginitis, urethritis, and nephritis.

Having mild diuretic and *kapha* reducing properties makes it valuable for cardiac edema and also helpful for breaking up and dispelling kidney stones. Its astringent properties act as a mild vasoconstrictor to the uterus, making it useful for painful and heavy menstruation.

Over consumption of this herb can have an irritating effect on the mucous membrane of the stomach, due its high tannin content. Therefore, it should be combined with other soothing demulcent herbs like licorice, *shatavari*, or marshmallow to help counter this.

When mixed with a small amount of fresh ginger, it can help to mitigate some of its *vata* provoking qualities as well. For sub-acute to chronic bladder infections, consider using its similar but gentler relative pipsissewa.

Uva ursi makes a nice sitz bath for the days following childbirth to relieve localized inflammation, sore perineal muscle, and to hasten the healing of vaginal tears. To prepare a sitz bath, boil 1/4 to 1/2 cup of the leaves in 1 gallon of water for 20 to 30 minutes and then add it to a tub of warm water. A tea of the leaves can also be used as a wash for treating minor cuts and rashes.

VALERIAN

Valerian spp.; Valerianaceae

TAGARA

Effect on Doshas: V- P+ K-
Rasa: bitter, pungent, sweet, astringent Virya: heating Vipak: pungent
Preparations: infusion, decoction, fresh or dried root tincture, medicated milk, essential oil.
Dosage: 1-9 g per day; tincture, 30-60 drops.

Parts used: rhizome.

Tissues: plasma, muscle, marrow and nerve.

Systems: nervous, digestive, respiratory, circulatory.

Properties: nervine, sedative, antispasmodic, analgesic, carminative.

Indications: cramps, spasms, colic, dysmenorrhea, flatulence, insomnia, hysteria, delirium, neuralgia, nervous tension and stress, vertigo, headaches, migraine, palpitation, epilepsy, convulsions, nervous cough, asthma, chronic skin conditions, tinnitus.

Precautions: high *pitta*, high doses may cause depression and melancholy.

Valerian is best known in both Ayurvedic and Western herbalism as a sedative herb with powerful antispasmodic properties. It has a grounding quality to the mobile or erratic quality of *vata* and a direct effect on the muscles and nervous system.

It is useful for treating high *vata* that has gone into the muscle tissue, which can be characterized by symptoms such as cramps, tics, tremors, spasms, and rigidity, as well as into the nervous system causing weakness, joint pain, tinnitus, vertigo, fainting, neuralgia, and a variety of neurological disorders. It is also used to ease uterine cramping as well as bronchial spasms during asthma attacks. For generalized musculoskeletal pain, it combines well with herbs like *ashwagandha* and *vidari*.

Valerian is commonly used to treat general stress and insomnia, although it can have a stimulating or heating effect on the mind, especially in *pitta* predominant individuals. Here it can be substituted for cooling nervine herbs like hops, skullcap, or *jatamansi*, which is one of its Indian relatives.

It effectively burns undigested toxins from the blood, joints, nerves, and colon and helps to relieve intestinal gas, bloating, and fermentation in the GI tract. The tea prepared from this herb is used in the treatment of pinworms and tapeworms. It is also used as an external application for treating eczema, ulcers, and other skin diseases.

Valerian is a valuable remedy for *vata* related headaches and headaches accompanied by shifting pain, nervous tension, anxiety, restlessness, and occipital pain due to constipation.

An effective sedative to induce a deep and sound sleep can be made by decocting 1 tsp. of the powdered root into a cup of whole milk and taken before bedtime.

For hypertension or neuromuscular pain caused by increased *vata*, it can be combined with *ashwagandha* in a ratio of 2 to 3.

Valerian essential oil can be applied to specific *marmas* (energy points) to calm *vata* disturbances of the muscles, nervous system, and the mind.

Tagara (*Valerian wallichi*) is the Eastern variety of the Western valerian. It is used in much the same way, but is not as dulling to the mind and body and is fairly *tridoshic* when used in moderation or along with more stimulating herbs like ginger, *ajwan*, or *vacha* (calamus). Another one of its relatives is the Ayurvedic herb *jatamansi* (*Nardostachys or Valeriana jatamansi*), which is a *sattwic* and *tridoshic* herb that has more of a rejuvenating effect upon the mind than either *tagara* or valerian.

VIDANGA

Embelia ribes; Myrsinaceae

Effect on Doshas: V- P+ K-
Rasa: pungent **Virya: heating** **Vipak: pungent**
Preparations: infusion, decoction, paste.
Dosage: 1-15 g per day.

Parts used: fruit, leaves, root, bark.

Tissues: plasma, blood, muscle, fat.

Systems: digestive, circulatory, urinary, respiratory, excretory.

Properties: alterative, carminative, expectorant, diuretic, anthelmintic, purgative, stimulant.

Indications: constipation, parasites, flatulence, abdominal distension and pain, yeast infections, candidiasis, hemorrhoids, fissure, fistula, diabetes, bronchial asthma, worms, fungal infections.

Precautions: high *pitta*, pregnancy.

Vidanga helps to do *mala shuddhi*, or cleansing of the waste products, hence it effectively rids the body of parasites, especially worms, from wherever they may be in the body. It pacifies both *vata* and *kapha*, increases *agni*, and is purifying to the liver, blood, lungs, and urinary tract.

As a carminative and digestive stimulant, it is effectively used in *vata* conditions accompanied by profuse *ama* in the colon, causing flatulence with an obnoxious odor. Whenever there are stinky, sticky feces, vidanga is the herb of choice to clean house.

From an Ayurvedic perspective, even excess candida, bacterial, and fungal infections are all born of *ama* and fall into the category of *krumi* (worms or parasites). In such conditions, vidanga gets to the root of the problem by helping to kindle the digestive fire, support liver function, and burn *ama* from the GI tract, thus helping to treat as well as prevent such conditions. For treatment of parasitical conditions of the blood, it combines well with *neem* and turmeric.

For treating children with worms, doses of 1/4 to 1/2 tsp. can be given with a little raw honey or sugar, administered twice daily, to kill and expel worms. A paste of the powdered herb is effective for treating ringworm and it can be combined with equal parts *neem*.

When mixed with turmeric and *shardunika*, it helps to control blood sugar levels and is used in the treatment of adult onset diabetes.

VIDARI-KANDA, VIDARI

Ipomoea digitata; Convolvulaceae

ALLIGATOR YAM, GIANT POTATO

Effect on Doshas: VP- K+
Rasa: sweet, bitter **Virya:** cooling **Vipak:** sweet
Preparations: infusion, decoction, medicated *ghee* or oil, milk decoction
Dosage: 3-15 g per day.

Parts used: tuberous root.

Tissues: works on all tissues.

Systems: nervous, digestive, circulatory, reproductive, urinary.

Properties: nutritive tonic, aphrodisiac, rejuvenative, alterative, diuretic, anti-inflammatory, antispasmodic, analgesic, nervine, demulcent, vulnerary.

Indications: infertility, impotency, dysmenorrhea, emaciation, general debility, ulcers, colitis, Crohn's disease, diarrhea, uterine cramping, hormonal imbalances, menopause, osteoporosis, frequent urination, chronic fatigue, hepatitis, enlargement of the liver and spleen, tachycardia, anorexia, weakness during pregnancy, enlarged prostate.

Precautions: high *kapha* and *ama* (in excess).

Vidari is frequently used in Ayurveda to rejuvenate the female reproductive system and it shares similar properties with wild yam (*Dioscorea villosa*). It helps to regulate the menstrual cycle, tone the uterus, nourish the ovum, and treat infertility, weakness during pregnancy, menopausal complaints, dysmenorrhea, menstrual cramping, and painful ovulation.

To promote lactation, 1 tsp. of the powdered herb can be boiled in a cup of milk and taken twice daily.

It is pacifying to both *vata* and *pitta* and has anabolic energy, helping to increase fat and muscle tissue. It improves the strength and tone of muscles and nerves and is used in the treatment of fibromyalgia, Parkinson's, chronic fatigue, muscle pain and weakness, tuberculosis, and to prevent emaciation.

For anorexia or bulimia, it can be given along with herbs like *jatamansi* to calm *vata* in the mind and nervous system. To treat frequent urination, it combines well with *ashwagandha* and *bala* to increase the tone of the urinary sphincter.

Vidari is a fine reproductive tonic for men and is effective in promoting spermatogenesis, especially when taken as a milk decoction. It also helps to treat enlarged prostate. For this, it can be combined with herbs like *ashwagandha*, kapi kacchu, *gokshura*, or saw palmetto.

It is extremely helpful to treat enlargement of the liver and spleen and other disorders of the liver and lymphoid tissue. For this, it is often mixed with herbs like gentian, *kutki*, barberry, turmeric, *kanchanar*, *neem*, and *guduchi*.

Vidari is a demulcent and mucilaginous substance, hence it helps to soothe inflammation of the GI tract and is useful to promote healing of peptic ulcers and ulcerative colitis. For irritable bowel related symptoms, such as alternating constipation and diarrhea, which is often associated with aggravated *vata* and *pitta doshas*, it combines well with herbs such as *shatavari*, *bilva*, licorice, and marshmallow.

Yerba Mansa

Anemopsis californica; Saururaceae

Effect on Doshas: V+ (in excess) PK-
Rasa: bitter, astringent Virya: heating Vipak: pungent
Preparations: infusion, decoction, tincture.
Dosage: 3-9 g per day; tincture, 20-60 drops.

Parts used: root, leaves.

Tissues: plasma, blood, fat.

Systems: lymphatic, urinary, digestive, respiratory.

Properties: antibiotic, antiseptic, anti-fungal, anti-inflammatory, astringent, carminative, anthelmintic.

Indications: infections, fungal infections, diarrhea, dysentery, giardia, candidiasis, pulmonary affections, digestive weakness, bacterial infections of the GI tract, gum disease, urinary tract infections, slow healing wounds, nausea, colitis, ulcers, catarrhal conditions.

Precautions: high *vata*.

Yerba mansa is a perennial flowering plant native to southwestern North America. It is pacifying to both *pitta* and *kapha* and helps to relieve inflammation of the mucous membranes of the GI tract, lungs, mouth, and urinary tract. It has natural antibiotic, anti-microbial, and antiseptic actions and is used in the treatment of upper respiratory tract infections, gastrointestinal ulcers, and ulcerative colitis.

Despite its anti-*pitta* action and bitter taste, it is considered to possess a mildly warming energy. It helps to clear congestion of mucous membranes and it works well when an inflammatory condition has continued into the subacute phase of an infection or injury, causing the cold and wet qualities of *kapha* to stagnate, thus slowing down the healing process.

Externally, it can be used as a tincture, tea, or ointment to promote healing of cuts, abrasions, and infections—especially fungal infections. The powdered root is a good remedy for athlete's foot.

Yerba mansa also helps to stimulate the excretion of nitrogenous wastes from the system and is beneficial for joint pains, including gout and other arthritic complaints.

Having astringent properties, the tea or diluted tincture can be used as a mouthwash for puffy, inflamed gums and combines well with bayberry, neem, echinacea, *bilva*, and prickly ash.

Yerba mansa also kindles the digestive fire, burns *ama*, and is effective for treating indigestion, intestinal infection, and giardia. It has similar actions to goldenseal and makes a good substitute for this endangered herb.

Traditional Herbal Preparations

Traditional Ayurvedic Formulas

In the classical texts there are references to many herbal compounds that have been used for hundreds if not thousands of years. They are typically mixtures of powdered herbs (churnas), but are made in tablet and pill form as well. Churnas are quick and easy to prepare and a very convenient way to administer medicine over extended periods of time. Churnas can be made into a tea or put directly in the mouth and washed down with water. Other ways include mixing then with other substances such as honey or ghee and eating them as a paste. Many of the compounds listed in this section are becoming more and more available in the West.

Ashwagandhadi Churna

Ingredients: Ashwagandha, vidari kanda.

Effect on doshas: V- P+ K+ (mildly and only in excess).

Dosage: 1-3 g. 2-3 times daily.

Precautions: high kapha and ama.

This is a vata pacifying compound and a rasayana to all bodily tissues, especially the muscle, nerve, and reproductive tissues. It is given to treat rheumatic and arthritic complaints, muscle wasting, and general debility, and is also used during convalescence. It has a calming effect and provides tone and strength to the nervous system. It relieves neuromuscular and arthritic pain and helps with insomnia and anxiety. As a reproductive tonic, it is commonly used for leucorrhea, impotence, nocturnal emissions, premature ejaculation, and enlarged prostate.

Avipattikara Churna

Ingredients: Triphala, trikatu, trivrit, clove, musta, vidanga, tejapatara, cardamom, nishotha, and rock candy.

Effect on doshas: VPK= balances all doshas.

Dosage: 1.5 to 3 g. 2-3 times daily.

Precautions: pregnancy

It is primarily used for pitta related digestive disorders such as amla pitta (sour pitta in the stomach), heartburn, vomiting, hyperacidity, gastritis, and irritable bowel syndrome. It has a purgative action to clear excess pitta from its main site, the small intestine. It also has carminative properties and is specific for sama pitta (pitta associated with ama). It helps to kindle agni, burn ama, and improve digestion. It is a nice formula for treating digestive disorders without aggravating pitta. Other uses of this formula include hemorrhoids, peptic ulcer, flatulence, abdominal discomfort, burning urination, and constipation.

Dashamula

Ingredients: Bilva, agnimantha, shyonaka, patala, kashimari, bruhati, kantakari, shalaparni, prushniparni, gokshura. (all root portions)

Dosha: V-P+ (in excess) K-

Dosage: powdered herb 1.5 to 3 g. 2-3 times daily.

Dashamula literally means "ten roots" and is used primarily to treat excess vata dosha characterized by debility. This compound nourishes and strengthens the muscles and calms and replenishes the nervous system. It is useful in the treatments of fatigue, poor digestive weakness, depression, anxiety, lingering fevers, tension headaches, tremors, Parkinson's disease, multiple sclerosis, as well as inflammatory conditions of the pelvic region including low back pain and sciatica. Dashamula also has a tonic effect on the lungs and is helpful for congestion, dry cough, and asthma. It can be taken in tea form or as a medicated wine (dashamula arista) for a fast acting and powerful effect. A strong decoction of the roots is commonly administered as a medicated enema to balance vata throughout the entire system, as well as to redirect apana vayu, the downward action of vata, thus cleansing and improving the tone of the colon.

Hingwashtak Churna

Ingredients: Black pepper, pippali, ginger, ajwan, rock salt, cumin, black cumin, and asafoetida (hing).

Effect on doshas: V- K- P+

Dosage: 1-3 g. twice daily.

Precautions: high pitta, pregnancy, diarrhea

Asafoetida (hing), which is a pungent and strong smelling resin, is the main herb in this compound. The primary action of this formula is on the GI tract and is used specifically to correct disorders of apana vayu, the downward moving aspect of vata that governs elimination. It is used to treat flatulence, bloating, hiccups, malabsorption, constipation, indigestion, parasites, low appetite, slow metabolism, and impacted wastes in the colon. Owing to its hot, pungent qualities, it is also pacifying to kapha. Although salt tends to increase kapha, in this formula it acts as a decongestive agent and helps to liquefy it.

Lavanbaskar Churna

Ingredients: Pippali, black pepper, 4 types of salt, ginger, and cardamom.

Effect on doshas: V- P+ K+

Dosage: 1-3 g. twice daily.

Primarily salty and pungent in taste, this formula is perfect for balancing samana vata and is used in a variety of vata types of digestive disorders, such as low appetite, constipation, indigestion, colic, flatulence, and sprue syndrome. It also helps to dissolve accumulations and obstructions due to excess kapha or ama.

Mahasudarshan Churna

Ingredients: Swertia chirata, triphala, trikatu, and many bitter herbs.

Effect on doshas: V+ P- K-

Dosage: 1-3 g. 2-3 times daily.

Precautions: pregnancy, high vata, emaciation.

This complex formula contains up to 40 herbs and is highly supportive to the immune system. It is a powerful antipyretic, antiviral, and diaphoretic used to burn ama and lower high fevers as in influenza and malaria. It is also given to treat disorders such as jaundice, nausea, gallstones, biliousness, hepatitis, cirrhosis, and enlargement of the liver and spleen. It helps to purify the blood and is used for a variety of infections, lymphatic congestion, and inflammatory disorders. Other uses of this medicine include dyspepsia, nausea, biliousness, allergies, asthma, bronchitis, sinus infections, abscess, mumps, anemia, lymphatic diseases, chronic fatigue, appendicitis, acne, skin diseases, eye diseases, and chronic inflammation of the eyelids.

Saraswati Churna

Ingredients: Vacha (calamus), ashwagandha, shankapushpi, ajwan, cumin, guduchi, bibhitaki, and fresh brahmi juice.

Effect on doshas: V- K- P+ (in excess).

Dosage: 1-3 g. 2-3 times daily.

Precautions: pregnancy, high pitta.

This compound is prepared with herbs that help to pacify and nourish the brain and nervous system. It is commonly used for treating vata related conditions such as mania, hysteria, epilepsy, anxiety, mental weakness, poor memory, speech disorders, and paralysis. It is also very effective for treating vata and kapha forms of depression.

Sitopaladi Churna

Ingredients: Vamsa rochana, pippali, cardamom, rock candy, and cinnamon.

Effect on doshas: VPK= balances all doshas.

Dosage: 1-3 g. 2-3 times daily.

This tasty formula helps to liquefy and expectorate kapha and phlegm while rejuvenating the lungs. It is mainly used to treat respiratory disorders such as sinus infections, cough, sore throat, bronchitis, asthma, fevers, and pleurisy. It also helps to burn ama, strengthen the digestive fire, and improve the appetite. One of the best ways to take this compound is as a warm tea with honey.

Talisadi Churna

Ingredients: Talisa, black pepper, ginger, pippali, vamsa rochana, cardamom, cinnamon, and rock candy.

Effect on doshas: V- K- P+ (in excess)

Dosage: 1-3 g. 2-3 times daily.

Precautions: high pitta.

This is a similar formula to Sitopaladi, but it also contains black pepper and talisa, so it is more heating and stimulating. It is used for treating vata and kapha related respiratory complaints, such as wet coughs and asthma. It helps to kindle the digestive fire and burn ama, and is also used for fevers, nausea, vomiting, malabsorption, emaciation, diarrhea, loss of appetite, and abdominal distention. Talisadi works well for coughs that linger after upper respiratory tract infections.

Trikatu Churna

Ingredients: Ginger, black pepper, and pippali.

Effect on doshas: V- P+ K- (may also increase vata in excess).

Dosage: 1-3 g. 2-3 times daily.

Precautions: high pitta, pregnancy.

This formula contains three pungent and heating herbs that kindle agni and burn ama, kapha, and fat. It helps to strengthen metabolic activity and is specific for treating kapha types of disorders. Because it is extremely hot, it can provoke pitta and in excess may aggravate the dry and light qualities of vata as well. It improves digestion, absorption, and assimilation of nutrients, and is commonly used for supporting weight loss. As an expectorant and bronchodilator, it is used for colds, coughs, wet forms of asthma, and congestive disorders. Other uses include obesity, malabsorption, food cravings, abdominal distention, and discomfort, fatigue, lethargy, high cholesterol, loss of appetite, parasites, and poor circulation.

Triphala Churna

Ingredients: Amalaki, bibhitaki, and haritaki.

Effect on doshas: VPK= balances all doshas.

Dosage: 1.5 to 3 g. 1-2 times dialy.

This is one of the most famous formulas in Ayurveda. It is a tridoshic, deep cleansing and rejuvenating tonic for the entire body. It is unique in that it helps to provide both a laxative as well as tonifying effect to the colon, thus regulating normal bowel function. It cleanses ama from the intestines and improves the tasks of all the organs of elimination. It is used to treat urinary, respiratory, and bowel diseases and is also given as a medicated ghee for many eye disorders. Triphala supports healthy respiratory, genitourinary, circulatory, and hepatic functions as well.

The ingredients are commonly used in equal proportions, but practitioners may add an extra part of one of the three to target a specific dosha. For example, amalaki for pitta, haritaki for vata, and bibhitaki for kapha disorders.

Medicated *Ghees*

Bitter Ghee (Tikta Ghritam, Maha Tikta Ghritam)

Tikta ghritam contains a variety of bitter herbs, including neem and guduchi, and is highly pitta pacifying. It is used to treat diseases of the liver and blood, as well as skin conditions such as acne, psoriasis, eczema, and leprosy. It has antiviral, anti-inflammatory, and antibiotic properties and helps to promote good cholesterol (HDL). Its action extends to majja dhatu (nerve tissue), so it can also be used to nourish and protect the nervous system in vata/pitta related afflictions such as multiple sclerosis. It can be used in a douche preparation by dissolving 1-3 tsp into warm water for relieving symptoms relating to vaginal yeast infections and leucorrhea.

Dosage: 1 to 3 tsp. twice daily with warm milk or water.

Brahmi Ghee (Brahmi Ghritam)

This ghee contains brahmi, shankapushpi and other herbs that calm and rejuvenate the mind and nervous system. It helps to pacify pitta and vata, and is used internally as well as in nasya (nasal therapy). Daily application of 3 to 5 drops of brahmi ghee to each nostril first thing in the morning on an empty stomach helps rejuvenate the mind. It can also be used to treat hoarseness of voice, memory loss, ADD, bipolar disorder, mania, epilepsy, insanity, migraine headaches, and many other mental disorders.

Dosage: 1 to 3 tsp. twice daily with warm milk or water.

Licorice Ghee (Yashti Ghritam)
Yashti ghritam soothes and pacifies vata and pitta throughout the entire GI tract. It can be used to calm inflammation and heal ulcers, including ulcerative colitis and peptic ulcers. Applied topically, it is also effective for treating diabetic ulcers and bedsores. For vata/pitta related gynecological conditions, such as cervical dysplasia, yeast infection, and interstitial cystitis, it can be applied to a tampon or in a douche of warm water.

Dosage: 1 to 3 tsp. twice daily with warm water or milk.

Shatavari Ghee (Shatavari Ghritam)
Shatavari ghee is commonly used to nourish arthava vaha srotas (female reproductive tissue) and rasa and rakta dhatus (plasma and blood tissues). It also pacifies pitta in all seven bodily tissues. Applied topically on the breasts, it promotes lactation and the health of the mastic tissue. Other uses include vaginal dryness, ulcers, menstrual disorders, menopausal symptoms, infertility, and hyper metabolic conditions. It can be taken internally and used topically, especially for vaginal dryness and breast massage. Pregnant women can massage it on the belly to prevent stretch marks and for its nourishing effects on the womb.

Dosage: 1 to 3 tsp. twice daily with warm water or milk.

Triphala Ghee (Triphala Ghritam, Maha Triphala Ghritam)
This ghee contains triphala, trikatu, and sandalwood, amongst other herbs. It is primarily used to treat various disorders of the eyes, including conjunctivitis, blepharitis, glaucoma, cataracts, and poor eyesight. It is also a rasayana to the entire GI tract and helps to protect ojas (vital essence and immunity). Plain triphala ghritam can be used for netra basti treatments, where ghee is used to bathe the eyes, and is very effective for eye disorders such as detached retina, uveitis, and diabetic retinopathy.

Dosage: 1 to 3 tsp. twice daily with warm milk.

Guggulu Preparations
A wide variety of herbal compounds are made along with guggulu (Commiphora mukul), many of which are used to treat vata disorders of the nervous system, arthritic conditions, and accumulations of excess kapha and ama. Aside from being a natural binding agent to form pills, guggulu is a yogavahi (catalytic agent) that helps to direct and enhance the actions of the herbs it is combined with.

Guggulu compounds are usually administered with other medicines, such as herbal infusions and decoction, to form a balanced and complete herbal program. For example, yogaraj guggulu is often given along with traditional herbal decoctions such as maharasnadi kvatha for conditions such as rheumatism and arthritis. Likewise, kaishore guggulu is given with mahamanjishthadi kvatha for skin diseases, gout, and other blood related disorders. Customized herbal formulas can also serve as a good foundation for treatment, whereas specific guggulu compounds can be chosen to target particular conditions.

Gokshuradi Guggulu

In this compound, guggulu serves as a catalyst for the herb gokshura, which is a rejuvenating tonic to the kidneys, urinary tract, and reproductive organs, especially the prostate. It also contains triphala and trikatu, which help to burn kapha and ama, thus detoxifying the entire genitourinary system. Gokshuradi guggulu is considered relatively tridoshic and is used to treat a wide variety of kidney, urinary, and reproductive complaints such as cystitis, urethritis, urinary stones, enlarged prostate, high cholesterol, polyuria, spermaturia, premature or painful ejaculation, incontinence, lumbago, and gout.

Dosage: 1-4 pills, 2-3 times daily.

Kaishore Guggulu

In this formula, the pitta pacifying herb guduchi plays a primary role. This compound is used to address conditions relating to excess pitta and ama in the joints, blood, muscle, and nerve tissue. It is commonly given to treat inflammatory types of arthritis as well as bursitis, tendonitis, gout, and fibromyalgia. It also helps to enhance metabolic functions, thus preventing further formation of ama, and to regulate thyroid activity. Other uses of kaishore guggulu include skin diseases, boils, acne, carpal tunnel syndrome, plantar fasciitis, bursitis, neuralgia, strained and sprained muscles, sciatica, myositis, dysmenorrhea, menorrhagia, headaches, lumbago, and rheumatism.

Dosage: 1-4 pills, 2-3 times daily.

Kanchanar Guggulu

This formula includes kanchanar, which is an herb specific for clearing accumulations of kapha and ama in the lymphatic and digestive systems. It also contains the compounds triphala, trijata, and trikatu to further help strengthen metabolic and eliminatory functions. Kanchanar guggulu is a key medicine in treating gandamala (swollen chain of lymph nodes in the neck), goiter, lymphatic and sinus congestion, cysts, fibroids, fistulas, edema, hemorrhoids, and benign tumors.

Dosage: 1-4 pills, 2-3 times daily.

Mahayogaraj Guggulu
This is a complex compound containing both herbal and mineral ingredients, including swarna bhasma (gold ash), which is highly effective for treating diseases affecting the nerve tissue such as epilepsy, paralysis, memory loss, and multiple sclerosis. It is also used for rheumatism, chronic and degenerative arthritis, heart disease, and occasionally for bronchitis and vata and kapha types of asthma.

Dosage: 1-3 pills, 2-3 times daily.

Punarnavadi Guggulu
This compound contains punarnava, a diuretic and demulcent herb, loha bhasma (iron ash), and guggulu, along with several other herbs. It is traditionally used to dispel excess kapha and ama via the urinary tract. It is helpful in disorders like obesity, edema, ascites, urinary tract ailments, urinary stones, gallstones, fibrocystic changes, high cholesterol, arteriosclerosis, hypertension, and lethargy. It is curative for kapha types of arthritis (characterized by stiff and swollen joints that are cool to the touch, achy in the morning and better with movement). Punarnava guggulu is also pacifying to pitta and is effective for treating jaundice, skin diseases, abscesses, and other inflammatory conditions. It has also proven to be beneficial as a cardiac tonic.

Dosage: 1-4 pills, 2-3 times daily.

Rasnadi Guggulu
This compound contains the herbs rasna, erandamula, devadaru, shunti (ginger), and guggulu and is used in conditions due to excess vata. It purifies the blood, effectively removes deposits of uric acid from the system, and is used in the long-term treatment of chronic or "old" gout. Rasnadi guggulu also relieves inflammation, pain, stiffness, and swelling associated with various arthritic complaints and helps to prevent joint degeneration.

Dosage: 1-3 pills, 2-3 times daily.

Simhanad Guggulu
This formula includes triphala, gandhak (sulphur), castor oil, and loha bhasma (iron ash). It pacifies vata and kapha, and burns and

eliminates ama from the joints, blood, and GI tract. It is one of the best medicines used in the treatment of ama vata (rheumatoid arthritis), especially in acute stáges and flare-ups, when vata is actively pushing ama into the joint spaces.

Dosage: 1-4 pills, 2-4 times daily.

Triphala Guggulu
Composed of triphala, trikatu, and guggulu and pontentized with a strong decoction (bhavana) of triphala, this guggulu compound is used to scrape away and remove ama and obstructions in the bodily tissues and channels. It kindles agni, especially in the meda dhatu (fat tissue), decreases ama in the GI tract, supports the metabolism, and is also helpful for controlling obesity. Its ability to prevent and rid the system of ama makes it a good medicine for boils, carbuncles, abscesses, allergies, toxemia, malabsorption, high cholesterol, hyperglycemia, and gallstones. Other uses include arthritis, fatigue, hypothyroidism, fistulas, constipation, hemorrhoids, sinus congestion, and rheumatism.

Dosage: 1-4 pills, 2-3 times daily.

Yogaraj Guggulu
This intricate formula contains nearly 20 herbs and is traditionally used to burn ama and manage excess vata and kapha. It has an affinity to the joints and is helpful in rheumatoid and osteoarthritis, and gout. It decreases excess vata in the joints and muscle tissue, characterized by popping, cracking joints or tics, tremors, spasms, lumbago, fibromyalgia, and so on. It also has a direct action upon the nerve tissue and is used in epilepsy, neuralgia, sciatica, and nervous debility. Other conditions related to excess vata that can be helped by this medicine are anemia, hearing loss, tinnitus, tingling and numbness, as well as vata types of heart, urinary, or reproductive conditions, including infertility.

Home Remedies & Kitchen Pharmacy

Many of the spices used in Indian and Ayurvedic cooking are also highly respected medicines that have played a key role in many traditional herbal compounds for thousands of years. The use of spices such as turmeric, cumin, fennel, coriander, and cardamom in the daily diet can have a significant impact on the prevention and management of disease, and also provide the six tastes (shad rasa) that are essential for proper digestion and nourishment. These spices can be made into home remedies for treating common ailments such as the flu, colds, digestive disorders, minor wounds, burns, headaches, constipation, fever, colic, and so on. Even today many families in India still rely on the inherited wisdom of using simple remedies to deal with day-to-day health disorders. Furthermore, some of these culinary herbs and spices can be of great benefit for even serious conditions such as diabetes and cardiovascular diseases.

Below is a list of common complaints and simple household remedies made up with easily available herbs, spices, and oils that can be safely used by the whole family. These remedies are not intended to take the place of constitutional treatment in the case of chronic or reoccurring disorders, but to help alleviate acute conditions and their symptoms.

Acne: Apply a little toothpaste to the pimple at night before bedtime.

Drink 1/4 to 1/2 cup aloe vera juice twice daily until acne improves.

A paste made with herbs such as turmeric, red or white sandalwood, and neem can be applied to the face for 1/2 hour daily.

Also, blend a cucumber and apply the paste the face and wash it off after 1/2 hour.

Seasonal Allergies: Take 1-2 tsp. fresh cilantro juice 2-3 times daily. Also, lubricate the nostrils with a small amount of ghee by placing a small amount of ghee on the pinky finger and inserting it into both nostrils. This helps to create a protective barrier against dusts and pollen.

For itchy and red eyes caused by allergies, rose water can be used as cooling eye drops.

Eat a small amount of local bee pollen daily. Increase the amount very slowly until you can eat as much as a teaspoon or so.

Arthritic Pain: Make an infusion with 1/2 tsp. dried ginger in 1 cup of hot water, add 1 tsp. castor oil, and take before bedtime. This can be taken daily to calm vata and burn and clear ama in the joint spaces and GI track.

Make an infusion with ½ to 1 tsp of turmeric powder and a pinch of fine ground black pepper powder in a cup of hot water and drink 2 twice daily. When arthitic pain is moderate to severe, I suggest using a standardized extract of turmeric in pill or capsule form.

Asthma: Make an infusion of 1 tsp. licorice powder in hot water and add 10 to 15 drops of mahanarayan oil. Stir well and take two sips every 5 to 10 minutes until the breathing improves.

For kapha types of asthma, characterized by difficult breathing and profuse mucus, the same method is used but with an infusion of equal parts licorice and ginger powder.

Also, drinking 1 cup of hot water before bedtime helps to relieve asthma symptoms.

Athlete's Foot: Soak feet in equal parts apple cider vinegar and water for a least 10 minutes daily until symptoms are gone.

Add 3 Tbsp. of baking soda per quart of water and soak the feet for a half hour daily. Cinnamon tea can also be used as an anti-fungal foot soak.

Powder the feet with baking soda before putting on socks and shoes. Wear open shoes as much as possible to keep the feet cool and dry.

Avoid wearing closed shoes whenever possible to allow the feet to get air and stay cool.

Bad Breath: Chew on the seeds of 1-2 pods of green cardamom after meals. A small amount of fennel seeds can also be chewed or added along with the cardamom.

It is also important to remember to scrape the tongue daily after brushing the teeth first thing in the morning.

Bleeding Cuts and Wounds: Apply ice to the affected area. Sandalwood paste or the ash of a burnt cotton ball or human hair can be also applied locally.

Applying corn starch, turmeric, or cayenne powder directly to minor wounds can also help to stop bleeding.

Boils: To bring a boil to a head, apply frequent warm water compresses to the site of the boil.

Make a paste with 2 parts steamed onion (made into a pulp) mixed with 1 part turmeric powder, apply it over the site of the boil, and wrap with gauze. Allow it to set for many hours or overnight and change it as needed until suppuration occurs. Internally, drink generous amounts of coriander tea at room temperature or slightly cooled.

Burns: If fresh aloe vera is available, filet a segment of the leaf, place it over the burn, and wrap with gauze to hold it in place.

A paste of fresh aloe pulp mixed with a pinch of turmeric can also help to relieve and heal minor burns. If fresh aloe is not available, then store bought aloe vera gel can be used.

A calendula salve or homeopathic gel should be kept in the house or first aid kit for this purpose. Rubbing a little cooking oil or ghee to the site of a burn helps to retain moisture in the tissue.

Canker Sores: Mix equal parts turmeric and honey or aloe juice and make a paste, which can be applied to the affected area, and repeat as needed. Also, rubbing a piece of onion directly on the canker helps to inhibit bacteria and promote healing.

Cavities (Prevention of): Chew on a cardamom pods daily after meals. Also, daily swishing with warm sesame oil helps to strengthen the teeth and gums. Chewing 1 heaping Tbsp. of white sesame seeds daily is a simple way of getting extra calcium.

Common Cold: A simple remedy for the common cold is warm ginger tea made with fresh or dried ginger.

Another good remedy is yogi tea, which is made with a 1-1/2 inch piece of fresh ginger root (chopped fine or grated), a stick of cinnamon, 1/2 tsp. licorice powder, and a few whole cloves boiled lightly in 1 quart of water for 10-15 minutes. This tea can be sweetened with raw honey once it has cooled down to drinking temperature.

Conjunctivitis: Apply a few drops of pure rose water into the eyes a few times a day. Turmeric tea is also very effective when used as eyewash. Prepare it by infusing 1 tsp. turmeric powder in 1 cup of room temperature water over night and then stain it through a coffee filter before using.

Another eyewash for conjunctivitis is diluted chamomile tea (cool). Simply place cotton balls soaked in the tea over the eyes.

Internally, a tea made from 1-2 tsp. of chamomile, coriander, or chrysanthemum flowers can be taken a few times a day.

Constipation: Simply drinking 1-2 glasses of warm water first thing in the morning can help to stimulate a bowel movement.

For mild constipation, mix 1-3 tsp. psyllium husk powder into a glass of water, stir, and drink before bedtime.

Warm milk is also a mild laxative. Heat 1 cup of milk, add 1-2 tsp. ghee and drink before bedtime. This can be used safely during pregnancy, whereas other laxatives are not recommended.

One of the best general bowel tonics and mild laxatives is triphala compound. For general use, mix 1/2 to 1 tsp. triphala into 1 cup of hot water, steep for 10-15 minutes, and drink before bedtime or early in the morning (5 am).

If there is dryness in the colon, characterized by hard, dry fecal matter, add 1 tsp. each of ghee and honey to a cup of triphala tea and take at bedtime.

For stubborn constipation, take 1 rounded tsp. of triphala and boil it for 5 minutes in a cup of water, strain, and drink before bedtime. For even a stronger laxative effect add 1-3 tsp. pure castor oil in a cup of ginger tea and drink before bedtime.

One of the best ways to increase dietary fiber is rink a fruit/ vegetable smoothie once a day.

Corns: Apply a small amount of castor oil to the corn and cover with a band-aid.

Cuts and Wounds: Apply raw honey to the affected area and cover. Honey is a remarkable remedy for cleansing the tissues as well as preventing and curing infections.

Cystitis and Burning Urination: Take 1 tsp. of freshly ground coriander seeds and steep in 1 cup of hot water. Let it cool and drink as often as needed.

Or mix a few drops of pure sandalwood oil into 1 tsp. raw sugar and eat it. This will cool down excess pitta quickly. Only do this if you have real sandalwood oil, not an artificial substitute.

Dehydration: Drinking a sugar and saline solution provides quick relief. Mix 1 tsp. sugar and a pinch or two of salt into a glass of room temperature water and drink as needed.

Diarrhea: Peel and dice two apples into medium size chunks, steam them until soft, and mash them into a sauce. Then add 1/8 tsp. (2 pinches) nutmeg and 1 tsp. ghee and stir together. This can be taken 1-2 times a day to help bind the stool.

Dizziness: Smelling a freshly chopped onion helps to provide circulation to the brain, thus providing instant relief.

Dry cough: Mix 1/2 tsp. turmeric powder and 1 tsp. turbinado sugar or raw honey, and eat 2-3 times a day.

Chew a small slice of fresh ginger dipped in sea salt.

Breathing steam from a bowl of hot water or the steam from a hot shower can help as well.

Also, mix 1/2 tsp. of sea salt into a cup of warm water and gargle as frequently as needed.

Earache: Wrap a small pinch of asafetida (hing) into a small piece of a cotton ball to form a small earplug and gently insert it into the ear.

Ear Infection: Three drops of garlic oil can be inserted into the ear for more moderate pain and mild infection.

Garlic mullein oil works best for ear infections and pain. This is a common blend that can be found at most health food stores.

Apply 1-3 drops of pure tea tree essential oil directly into the ear 1-2 times daily.

Applying a warm compress to the ear helps to bring circulation and provides pain relief.

Fatigue (General or Chronic): Place thirty pitted dates and fill a quart size mason jar. Cover the dates with melted ghee, let it cool completely, and cap the jar. Store it for one month and then eat 1 date each morning for one month or longer.

Fever: To help break a fever, especially during the flu, steep 1 tsp. tulsi and 1 tsp. freshly shredded ginger in 1 cup of hot water for 15 minutes, strain and drink before bedtime. Regular basil can be used as a substitute, if tulsi (holy basil) is not available.

Topically, the fresh juice of an onion can be applied to the navel region to lower high fevers. This is a good remedy for infants and young children. To make the juice, dice 1/2 an onion and blend in a blender with a little water, then strain and apply.

Fungal Infections of the Nails: Stir 1/2 a tsp. turmeric into a tablespoon of coconut oil and apply to the affected nail and wrap with a band-aid. This is not a quick treatment but it works. The most effective way to allow the turmeric to penetrate under the nail is to use a alcohol based turmeric tincture, which is also less messy than the oil method.

Gas and Bloating: Mix 1 tsp. fennel seeds (whole or powdered) with 1 tsp. freshly shredded ginger and 1/4 tsp. ground cardamom seeds into a cup of hot water and let it steep until drinking temperature.

Another simple remedy consists in steeping 1/2 to 1 tsp. ajwan powder in a hot cup of water or ginger tea and drinking before or after food.

For sluggish digestion, mix 1 Tbsp. each of cumin, coriander, and cumin seeds to 1 quart of water. Bring to a boil and then simmer for 10 minutes. Drink throughout the day.

A good Ayurvedic compound to keep around the kitchen for occasional gas, poor appetite, and weak digestion is hingwashtak churna. This can be taken in 1/2 tsp. size doses with warm water before food.

Gastritis or Peptic Ulcer: Make an infusion of 1/2 tsp. licorice and 1/2 tsp. shatavari in 1 cup of water and take 2-3 times daily after meals.

Also, in the case of ulcers, mix enough arrowroot powder with milk to form a pudding and eat it in small amounts a couple times daily until the ulcer is healed. This can promote healing of ulcerative colitis as well.

Eating one banana daily has proven quite useful for healing peptic ulcers. Other remedies include drinking homemade almond milk or fenugreek (methi) tea made with the powdered seeds.

Gum problems: For puffy, bleeding, or receeding gums, add a few drops of pure tea tree oil into a glass of water and gargle several times daily.

Massage the gums firmly with coconut oil infused with a few drops of tea tree oil.

Hair Loss: Massage the scalp vigorously with almond, sesame, or coconut oil daily, before bedtime. Neem oil is also very beneficial for strenghtneing the roots of the hair.

Rinse the scalp with several cups of triphala tea (strained) and let it remain in the hair for 1/2 to 1 hour. Nettle tea is also good as an herbal rinse.

Add a 3-4 Tbsps. apple cider vinegar to a quart of water, rinse the hair, and let it sit for a few hours before washing it off.

Add 10-15 drops of tea tree essential oil to the amount of shampoo you use to wash your hair.

Headaches: For occipital headache, often related to constipation, apply a drop of nutmeg oil on the temples. Here, triphala tea should be taken daily at bedtime.

Also, make a fine ginger paste and apply it to the forehead and allow it to set and dry. For sinus headaches, this ginger paste can be applied over the maxillary sinuses as well.

If headaches are caused by excess pitta, then pure sandalwood or khus oil or paste can be applied to the temples and third eye. Drinking coriander tea is helpful to remove excess heat from the body.

Hemorrhoids: Add 1/2 tsp. turmeric into1 tsp. ghee or coconut oil to make a paste and apply topically to the hemorrhoids. Applying castor oil can help to relieve irritation and inflammation as well. Avoid wiping with dry toilet paper.

Hiccups: Suck on or chew a small piece of fresh ginger and wash it down with a little warm water.

Mix together 1 tsp. castor oil and 1/2 tsp. honey and lick some every few minutes until hiccups improve.

Eat fresh yogurt with 1-2 tsp. sea salt.

High Cholesterol: Soak 1 tsp. fenugreek seeds in 1 cup of water overnight. Strain the tea and drink it, first thing in the morning.

Another remedy is to mix 1 tsp. each of fresh grated ginger and minced garlic, 1 tsp. lime juice, and a pinch of sea or rock salt, and eat before or after a meal.

Hoarseness: A mixture made from 1/4 tsp. black pepper and 1 tsp. honey can be sucked on to nourish the throat and improve the voice.

Gargle with a mixture of a 1/2 tsp. sea salt into 1 cup of warm water.

Hyperacidity: Mix a 1/4 tsp. baking soda into 1/2 cup of yogurt and eat 1 hour before mealtime.

Mix 1/4 tsp. baking soda into a 1/2 cup of warm water, add 10 drops of fresh lime juice, and drink.

Insomnia: Add 1/8 tsp. nutmeg to 1 cup of hot milk and take before bedtime. If this doesn't work, then a stronger approach may be necessary to calm vata by making an infusion of 1 tsp. ashwagandha and 1/2 tsp. tagar (or valerian).

Garlic milk is also used to induce a sound sleep, especially when vata is the cause. Boil 1 clove of garlic (chopped) in a cup of milk for 5 minutes, strain, and drink before bedtime.

For topical use, mix a few pinches of nutmeg powder into a small amount of ghee and apply it around the eye sockets and temples before bedtime. This helps with vata type of headaches as well.

Massaging the scalp and soles of the feet with a little warm sesame oil before bedtime helps to calm the mind. For pitta types, bhringaraj or coconut oil can be used instead of plain sesame oil.

Ayurveda recommends a short passive meditation before sleep to calm the mind and help let go of the day.

Jet Lag: Drink a cup of ginger tea, or take 1-2 "00" size ginger capsules before and after flying.

Low Appetite: Chew a small slice of fresh, peeled ginger dipped into mineral or sea salt before a meal and wash it down with a little warm water.

Low Sexual Energy: Drink 1 cup of warm milk with a pinch of saffron at bedtime.

Another remedy consists in boiling 1 tsp. ashwagandha or shatavari in 1 cup of milk and 1/2 cup of water until 1 cup liquid remains. This can be taken first thing in the morning or at bedtime.

Blend 10 soaked, peeled almonds, 2-3 fresh dates (soaked and pitted) into 1 cup of milk or water along with a pinch of saffron and cardamom and drink.

Add foods such as milk, avocados, apples, figs, almonds, bananas, persimmons, eggs, onions, garlic, and celery to your diet.

Menstrual Cramps: Combine a 1/4 tsp. black pepper or ginger powder into 1/4 cup of aloe vera juice and drink 2-3 times a day, or as needed.

Muscle Aches: Add 1/2 a cup each of sea salt (or powdered ginger) and baking soda to a hot tub and soak for 15-30 minutes.

Muscle Cramps: Dip a towel into a pot of hot ginger tea, ring it out, and apply as a fomentation to the affected area.

Another approach is to massage mahanarayan, sesame, or mustard oil into the affected area and then take a warm bath in a tub infused with 1/2-cup each of ginger powder (or sea salt) and baking soda, and sit for 15-30 minutes. This is best done before bedtime.

Nausea: Steep 1 tsp. fennel powder into 1 cup of hot water and drink a few times a day. Fresh ginger tea with fennel is also helpful.

Ginger in almost any form is a sovereign remedy for nausea. It can be made as a tea in either its fresh or dried form or taken in capsule form. Old fashion ginger ale and even ginger candy can be helpful to calm the belly.

Steep 1 tsp. or one teabag of peppermint or chamomile in a cup of hot water and drink.

Poisoning (Chemical): Do not induce vomiting. Drink 1 cup of milk or a medium strength cup of licorice tea with 1-2 tsp. ghee added to it, and seek immediate medical attention.

Rashes: Blend 1 cup of fresh cilantro leaves in a blender with just enough water to make a semi-thick paste, then apply the paste to the affected area. Fresh cilantro is one of the best home remedies for cooling the blood and relieving hot itchy rashes such as hives, poison ivy, and so on.

Also, cilantro juice can be squeezed out from the pulp and gently rubbed onto the rash and left to dry. This is a convenient method and less messy than using the paste.

Fresh cilantro juice can also be taken internally in 1-2 tsp. size doses along with room temperature coriander tea (1 tsp. per cup of water), 2-3 times daily.

Sinus Congestion: Combine equal parts licorice and ginger powder, and add 1 tsp. of this mixture to 1 cup of hot water. When the tea becomes drinking temperature, add 1 tsp. raw honey (never add honey to boiling water, as it will promote toxicity). This can be taken 3 times a day.

To relieve headaches due to sinus congestion, make a paste from dried ginger powder (or cinnamon) and apply to the forehead. Be careful as to avoid any of it going into the eyes. Allow the paste to sit until dry, then carefully remove it with a face cloth.

Drinking tulsi tea on a daily basis is a good habit for those prone to sinus congestion due to allergies. Other common herbs and spices for relieving sinus congestion include mullein, fenugreek, black pepper, and tulsi.

Sore Throat: Mix 1 tsp. turmeric powder and 1/2 tsp. sea salt in a cup of warm water, and gargle as often as needed to relieve sore throat during a cold or flu. People with the tendency to suffer from sore throat and strep throat can also use this gargle regularly, as a preventative measure.

Strains and Sprains: Apply a warm paste made from 1 part ginger and sea salt, and 1/2 part turmeric mixed together with just enough warm water to make a paste. Spread the paste locally and wrap carefully with thick gauze. Change twice daily.

Salt and soda baths can also be helpful, or massaging with warming massage oils, like sesame, almond, mustard, or mahanarayan.

A simple pain relieving oil can be made by pressing 2 tsp. of the fresh juice from finely shredded ginger into sesame oil and used to massage sore joints and muscles.

Ayurveda does not recommend ice therapy for sprains after the first twenty four hours. If ice is used, it should be contrasted with warmth, as with a warm towel foot bath or hot water bottle, to promote circulation.

Toothache: Apply clove oil to the sore tooth to relieve the pain.

Warts: Turmeric and aloe can be made into a thin paste and applied to the warts. This can also be used for vaginal warts.

Thuja essential oil can be applied topically to warts 2-3 times daily and kept covered with a band-aid. This is the most effective external method for removing warts that I know of. This oil is toxic when taken internally or applied to large areas of the body, so use with caution.

Wrist Pain: Fill a kitchen sink with hot water and add in 1/4 cup of fresh ground brown or yellow mustard seeds and soak your tired arms and hands for 5-10 minutes. Repeat as needed.

Botanical Index

A

B

C

D

L

M

N

O

P

R

S

T

U

V

W

Y

Index

A

B

D

E

F

G

H

L

M

N

R

S

T

U

V

W

Y

AYURVEDA HEALTH & WELLNESS SERIES

General Editor : ***Dr. David Frawley***

Editorial Board :

Dr. Shekhar Annambhotla, Dr. Sunil V. Joshi, Dr. Suhas G. Kshirsagar, Dr. G.C. Jain

1. **The Ayurvedic Diet:** ***The Ancient Way to Health Rejuvenation and Weight Control***—DENNIS THOMPSON [978-81-7822-014-7] ₹ **350**
2. **Tibetan Ayurveda**—ROBERT SACHS [978-81-7822-327-8] ₹ **295**
3. **Vedic Health Care System**—RAM LAL SHAH, BINOD KUMAR JOSHI & OTHERS [978-81-7822-041-5] ₹ **225**
4. **Neti**—DAVID FRAWLEY [978-81-7822-299-X] ₹ **350**
5. **Ayurvedic Healing**—DAVID FRAWLEY [978-81-208-0957-4] (C) ₹ **495**
   [978-81-208-1003-7] (P) ₹ **350**
6. **Soma in Yoga and Ayurveda**—DAVID FRAWLEY [978-81-208-3630-3] (P) ₹ **395**

YOG TRADITION OF INDIA

Editorial Board:

Dr. Jitendra B. Shah, Dr. S. F. Biria, Prashant S. Iyengar

An anthology of the discourses were expounded by Prashant Iyengar for the students, scholars and sadhakas of Yog at different points of time, presented here in the form of books. The engaging style of narration will appeal to the readers' brain and heart while they imbibe the knowledge of Yog, For easy comprehension, the words in the Sandhis are separated in the Sanskrit quatation. The books selected to be published under the series are:

1. **Ashtanga Yoga of Patanjali:** *Philosophy, Religion, Culture, Ethos and Practices —Prashant S. Iyengar* [978-81-7822-480-0] ₹ **750**
2. **Discourses on Yog**—*Prashant S. Iyengar* [978-81-7822-481-7] ₹ **500**
3. **A Manual on Humanics**—*Prashant S. Iyengar* [978-81-7822-479-4] ₹ **200**
4. **Pranayama:** *A Classical and Traditional Approach —Prashant S. Iyengar* [978-81-7822-482-4] ₹ **400**